Handbook of Medical Law and Ethics for Nurses

Handbook of Medical Law and Ethics for Nurses

MARK W. GIBSON, LLM, B.Sc (Hons), RMN, RGN, LPE, Dip.Mgmt
Independent Scholar
York, England, United Kingdom

ELSEVIER

ISBN: 978-0-7020-8354-9
Printed in Poland
Last digit is the print number: 9   8   7   6   5   4   3   2   1

Content Strategist: Robert Edwards
Content Project Manager: Arindam Banerjee
Design: Ryan Cook
Marketing Manager: Deborah Watkins

CONTENTS

Over time, the practice and related theory of nursing have become more technical, with an increasing emphasis on the importance of bonding clinical practice to a sound knowledge base. In striving to achieve this, the need for the nurse to place the safety and welfare of the patient at the core of their decisions and actions remains as convincing as ever, and helps develop a greater appreciation of the legal implications of being a 'professional' nurse. Indeed, the author's interest in matters of law concerning medicine and healthcare stems from their own past experience of monitoring, managing and learning from patient safety incidents. This handbook is aimed at the nurse—clinician or manager—who requires a concise, easy-to-read reference source that can assist them in the course of their work duties. Moreover, if the book quenches the reader's thirst to engage in further study on law and ethics, then it is hoped that this text may provide the nurse a springboard toward future career enhancement, as well as enabling them to be more informed as a practitioner. Therefore, any further knowledge that this book brings to the nurse is intended to assist with both effective clinical decision-making and enhancing reflection on practice.

Public expectations of the professional health worker's duty of care, as well as the regulation of healthcare professionals serving to ensure the safety of the public as healthcare service users, remains high. This, consequently, enables patients to be confident in raising concerns and seeking advocacy within a legal system that works with the patient to pursue better care and gain fair and just access to processes in resolving matters of dispute and negligence claims. However, for many nurses, law and ethics has often featured during their career as a side subject, something to be 'dipped' into only when required. Nevertheless, over recent years, the accumulation of healthcare governance, the Human Rights Act 1998, high media profile court cases, public enquiries and the influence of the service-user movement has resulted in matters of law and ethics gaining a higher profile. This is none such than in cases where persons have suffered serious injury or death as a result of a failure in the provision of healthcare. With the raised expectations of the public regarding healthcare service provision, the professional nurse who values their autonomy as a clinical practitioner has raised the focus on their level of accountability, as required with the increasing responsibility that such autonomy brings.

Mark W. Gibson

Abortion Regulations 1991
Access to Medical Reports Act 1988
Abortion Act 1967 (as amended by Section 37 of the Human Fertilisation and
    Embryology Act 1990)
Abortion (Northern Ireland) Regulations 2020
Adoption and Children Act 2002
Adults with Incapacity (Scotland) Act 2000
Births and Deaths Registration Act 1953
Care Standards Act 2000
Children Act 2004
Children Act 1989
Civil Evidence Act 1972
Coroner and Justice Act 2009
Courts and Crime Act 2013
Damages Act 1996
Damages (Personal Injury) Order 2001
Data Protection Act 2018
Defamation Act 2013
Disability Discrimination Act 1995
Employment Rights Act 1996
European Communities Act 1972
Equality Act 2010
Family Law Act 1996
Family Law Reform Act 1987
Freedom of Information Act 2000
General Data Protection Regulation (including Data Protection Act 2018)
Gender Recognition Act 2004 (UK) Section 22
Gender Recognition (Disclosure of Information) (England, Wales and Northern
    Ireland) Order 2005
Gender Recognition (Disclosure of Information) (Scotland) Order 2005
Health and Social Care Act 2012
Health and Safety at Work etc. Act 1974
Health and Safety at Work Act 1974
Health and Social Care Act 2008
Health and Social Care Act 2008 (Regulated Activities) Regulations 2014
Health and Social Care (Safety and Quality) Act 2015 (England)
Health Service (Control of Patient Information) Regulations 2002
Health Professions Order 2001
Human Fertilisation and Embryology Act 1990 (UK) Section 33A
Human Rights Act 1998

This book is dedicated to all those, past and present, who work in the NHS with compassion, commitment and determination that often goes above and beyond public expectations.

Introduction to Law and Ethics

KEY TERMS

Criminal law
Civil law

Ethics
Professional values

Introduction

Most people are accustomed from their own early years and the years leading to adulthood of parentally imposed 'rules' imbedded in their consciousness as they develop and grow up. In abiding by such rules, they experience what they are allowed to do but also what they should not do. Therefore, as people mature and develop, they conform with the rules, influenced by their respect and affection for their parents or guardians as well as their perception of authority. Conversely, their understanding and possible fear of the adverse consequences of breaking those rules also plays a major influence. Thus, as people mentally develop and come of age, they may attain some moral ('good' or 'bad' or 'right' and 'wrong') values which are influenced by a number of factors, such as cultural norms, thus developing a lifestyle of adhering to societal rules, which are often based upon particular principles. Conversely, people may depart from the behavioural norms expected from following such principles, and thus 'break' the rules.

Law: Background

In making the distinction between 'rules' and 'law', law is principally the 'body of rules enacted or customary in a community and recognised as enjoining or prohibiting certain actions and enforced by the imposition of penalties' (Oxford Dictionaries, 2011). Therefore, departing from the norms and body of rules may well have consequences for those who breach such, and such rules function in the United Kingdom within a foundation of regulation and legislation normally confined to Acts of Parliament and those powers (i.e. to enforce the 'law') conferred by such Acts.

Currently, English law exists as a set of rules resulting from common law and statute by which people live their lives. The *common law* originates from the royal courts and has existed approximately since the year 1307; it has steadily evolved throughout history, as new cases have arisen. It is often regarded as a 'judge-made' law, serving as a yardstick and applied by the courts. A court is 'a body established by law for the administration of justice by "judges" and "magistrates"' (Oxford Dictionary of Law, 2018). Common law decisions are recognised as 'case law' and as such can form the benchmark for decision making in future cases. Examples include the 'Bolam Test' (*Bolam v Friern HMC*) and the 'Neighbour Principle' (*Donoghue v Stevenson*), which remain influential within the UK civil courts (detailed later in this book) and form a principle of law known as 'precedent', which serves as an authority for reaching the same decision in subsequent cases, and that facts of later cases are similar to those of the previous case (Oxford Dictionary of Law, 2018). Conversely, *Statutory Law* (Legislative Law) is that aspect of law which is enacted by Parliament in the working together of the House of Lords and House of Commons – written law and for a scripted piece of UK legislation to become an Act of Parliament, it must receive agreement of the Crown through Royal Assent. Examples of statutory law are The Health and Safety at Work Act 1974, The Equality Act 2010, the National Health Service and Community Care Act 1990 and the Data Protection Act 1998. Statutes are the highest mode of law and can upturn common law (e.g. abolition of the death sentence); however, common law cannot upturn statutory law. Indeed, Parliament may abolish previous statutes to bring in new legislation if it considers it essential. Such legislation comes under the umbrella of primary law. Under secondary law, sources such as Parliamentary white papers setting out major policy proposals, draft Acts of Parliament (bills), Parliamentary select committee reports e.g. debates, government guidance, Codes of Practice and textbooks/websites are included. Secondary law is not binding upon judges in the same way as a legislation or case law.

Criminal and Civil Law – What's the Difference?

Criminal law can be regarded as public law which governs relations of people as citizens of the state, whereas civil law is private law which is that part of law which governs relations of citizens among themselves. Under criminal law, if someone is found guilty of an offence, then it will result in an imposition by the State of some form of punishment (e.g. a fine, community service or a custodial sentence). Civil law concerns issues related to aggrieved persons (claimants) intending to seek some form of compensation (usually financial) in the form of damages as a remedy for the loss or harm suffered by an individual or 'corporate persons' such as an National Health Service (NHS) Trust, Health Authority, or private healthcare provider. As succinctly explained by Geldart (1996) 'the difference between civil law and criminal law turns on the difference between two different objects which law seeks to pursue – redress or punishment'. In other words, civil law seeks to achieve a remedy for the injured party and criminal law seeks to punish for an offence. The UK legal system is based upon the foundation that the accused is innocent unless proved to be guilty, hence, the burden of proof is on the person making the allegation, for example, a healthcare user wishing to claim compensation for damages against a hospital that they have accused of a wrongdoing which has caused injury. Specifically, the burden of proof in criminal law lies upon the prosecution (Crown) to prove their case *beyond reasonable doubt*, which means that the judge and/or jury must be satisfied by at least 95% or more that the accused is guilty of the charge. As this is a high standard of proof, where any reasonable doubt may lead to an acquittal of the charge, the difficulty of achieving this high standard can lead the Crown Prosecution Service (CPS) only to proceed if there is ample evidence for a conviction. In civil law the standard of proof is on the *balance of probabilities* and the burden upon the claimant to prove 51% or more that their case is more probable than not; that is, the defendant is liable for the loss, damage or harm. For a brief overview, see Table 1.1 (below).

Nevertheless, it is possible for a defendant to be acquitted (i.e. 'not guilty'), for example, in a manslaughter charge in a criminal trial, but held to be liable in a Civil Court, as the level of proof in civil matters is lower and thus, easier to achieve. Even though the possibility of facing a civil action is greater than a criminal

TABLE 1.1 ■ **Key Differences Between Criminal Law and Civil Law**

	Criminal Law	**Civil Law**
Meaning	Safety and protection of people and protection and regulating behaviour as offences against the public	Defines the private rights and responsibilities of persons and governs the relationship between persons
Action	Offences against the state, the person or property	Contract; property; company; family or Tort of negligence; defamation; nuisance; trespass and false imprisonment
Penalties	Fines; imprisonment; community service orders	Compensation; specific performance i.e. fulfilment of contractual obligations; injunctions; rescission
Standard of proof	Beyond all reasonable doubt	Balance of probabilities
Burden of proof	Crown prosecution	Claimant

charge, cases of gross medical negligence (e.g. an allegation of manslaughter) would be tried in a court under the jurisdiction of Criminal Law. Consequently, both criminal and civil law can overlap, as the case of *R v Adamako* illustrates (see Case Study 1.1).

CASE STUDY 1.1   **R v Adomako [1995] 1 AC 171**

An anaesthetist, Mr Adomako (the defendant) was carrying out his responsibilities during an eye operation, for which it was necessary to place the patient under a general anaesthetic. During the operation and whilst under Mr Adomako's supervision, an endotracheal tube (connected to his oxygen supply) became disconnected from the ventilator and the patient suffered a fatal cardiac arrest. Mr Adomako was convicted of manslaughter by breach of duty. Mr Adomako questioned the legal basis of involuntary manslaughter by breach of duty and appealed the conviction.

Mr Adomako's appeal was dismissed and it was held that in cases of manslaughter by criminal negligence involving a breach of duty, the ordinary principles of the law of negligence applied to determine whether he had been in breach of a duty of care. Upon establishing the said breach, the question was of establishing causation and if this could be so established, whether it should be characterised as gross negligence and consequently, a crime. Ultimately, this was a question for the jury, with regard to the risk of the death concerned, asking themselves 'was the defendant's conduct so bad in all the circumstances that it ought to amount to criminal?'

Medical Law and Ethics

Medical law can be regarded as the most recent arm of civil law with its own sphere of legal study and research, and as Brazier and Cave (2016) have noted, 'The law's relationship with medicine has become a highly publicised affair. Rarely a day passes without media coverage of some new controversy surrounding medical practice, or medical ethics'. Medical law is made up of parts from the wider field of law, but mainly that of tort law. A 'tort' is 'a wrongful act or omission for which damages can be obtained in a civil court by the person wronged, other than a wrong that is only a breach of contract' (Oxford Dictionary of Law, 2018). In parallel with the growth of this new legal area is a political shift of power where 'medical paternalism no longer rules', as noted in the case of *Chester v Afshar*. This referred to the historic notion that 'medical decisions were regarded as clinical matters best reached by the experts and anyone seeking to challenge a doctor's decision in the court faced an uphill struggle' (Herring, 2020). Courts are more willing to challenge medical decisions and be involved in resolving complex ethical dilemmas concerning patients. This trend of moving the power away from doctors (and the 'caring' professions of nurses and Allied Health Professionals) was asserted in the NHS Constitution 2013, which lists the rights of patients and states that services should be 'patient-led', where 'The patient will be at the heart of everything the NHS does' (NHS, 2013).

Perhaps a subject more difficult to define than law is ethics. A dictionary definition of *ethics* is of 'moral principles that govern a person's behaviour or the conducting of an activity' (Concise Oxford English Dictionary, 12th ed). An example of such an 'activity' is that of the practice of nursing. 'Ethics' is derived from the Greek word *ethos,* meaning 'custom', 'habit', 'character' or 'disposition', and the term 'morals' is derived from the Latin word *moralis,* meaning 'manner', 'way' or 'custom'. Hence, ethics is a system of moral principles that lean towards a person's decisions and are of a more subjective understanding of 'right' and 'wrong' by a person. Conversely, morals emphasise the commonly shared societal norms about 'right' and 'wrong', but may be influenced by religion, family and education; for example, opinions influencing end-of-life decisions or abortion. 'Medical ethics is the application of ethical reasoning to medical decision-making' (Somerville, 2003). Thus, ethics applied to nursing care is the application of such reasoning to the holistic needs of the patient, and as highlighted by Wheeler (2012), 'Moral values guide our thinking and behaviour and impact on our ethical decision-making in relation to caring'. Law and ethics co-exist. If *law* is aimed at maintaining social order, *ethics* can be regarded as a code of moral behaviour that implies an intention of improving the person, such as establishing altruistic behaviour. Such moral behaviour is often unwritten, whereas law is presented in a written form (i.e. legislation). Thus, ethics implies an obligation of one person to another; it is linked to law in that law often has a foundation of moral values such as honesty, fairness and justice. For example, is the motorist who drives their car at 25mph in a 30mph zone doing so because they are considerate and aware of the safety of others by reducing the risk of an accident? Or perhaps it is because they are being followed by a police vehicle and might be at risk of receiving a fine and penalty points; additionally, it could be a combination of both – lawful and morally correct!

In order to gain a better understanding, a further breakdown of a system of ethics is that of two main types – normative and non-normative. Normative ethics looks at the norms and principles used by people when they make moral choices or decisions, and it questions the duties or values underpinning moral choices (Thompson, 2019). It questions what a person 'ought to do' in terms of their duties and involves the application of protocols, theories, rules, concepts and principles to professional practice – standards of 'right' or 'good' action. Two types of non-normative ethics are present – descriptive ethics and meta-ethics, both of which 'aim to identify what morality "is" rather than what ought to be' (Beauchamp and Childress, 2013). Descriptive ethics relates to what a person does and effectively examines moral beliefs, values and conduct and how a person thinks and behaves within a particular culture or social group. On the other hand, meta-ethics deliberates over moral language to establish the meaning and foundation of terms such as *values, morality, rights* and *obligation.* For example, in questioning such moral 'language' it would question the commonly used term *good* and/or *goodness.* Seedhouse (1998) gives a concise explanation of the meaning of the term 'good' in that it can be a description of objects that are useful; a description of things that themselves are pleasing or enjoyable; and a description of that which is specifically moral, that is, using words such as 'just' or 'right'. Therefore, meta-ethics considers the context of such language, and in the domain of clinical care, the question could be raised of what makes a good nurse.

The Influence of Professional Values

Values are fundamental beliefs which guide our motivations and actions. A value is defined as 'The worth, desirability, or utility of a thing, or the qualities on which these depend...' (Oxford Dictionaries, 2011). Hence, values are the personal and professional qualities a person chooses to interpret the world and also to guide their actions – being the sort of person they want to be, and the manner in which they treat themselves and others. Even though a person's values may be about what they regard as 'good/bad', 'right/wrong', desirable or worthwhile, then, such values may not necessarily be moral. Thus, within clinical practice, pursuing the beliefs of one's own professional values may not always guarantee being ethically sound, as what one healthcare professional values in a particular clinical situation may be different from the beliefs and values of another healthcare professional within the same situation. As there are occasions when a person's own values determine their attitude towards certain issues and the sort of person they are, and why they respond to people and events in their life as they do, Elcock et al. (2019) make note of a resulting potential dissonance within the professional context. They explain that the person (as 'nurse'), in adopting the professional values of the organisation they work for, should be aware of their own values, beliefs and attitudes, as these may vary from the NHS and organisational standards that must be followed in professional practice (Elcock et al., 2019). This perspective conveys the assumption that the nurse, during the course of their duties, needs to be mindful of their own responsibility to self-manage the interaction of values, professional standards and ethical behaviour that occurs within a complex framework of legal regulation.

Professional nursing values form an integral component of a healthcare provider organisation's overall assumed framework of values. Such organisational values were placed under in-depth scrutiny from 2010 to 2013 as part of the Mid Staffordshire NHS Foundation Trust Public Enquiry, culminating in the Francis report (Francis, 2013), which referred to a failure to protect patients from unacceptable risks described by Holmes (2013) as a 'profound crisis of culture at every level of the health service', where a number of failings in patient care resulted in preventable suffering and an abnormally high mortality rate. The professional principles of the values of caring had declined, and in many cases had been absent where it was stated that an overall picture of the Mid Staffordshire hospitals was that of '...a Trust devoid of humanity, totally incapable of recognising patients as people' (Holmes, 2013).

This financially costly enquiry produced over a million pages of evidence, including witness statements from patients, hospital staff, board members, ministers and senior civil servants. The sphere of the enquiry extended to determining what the regulatory bodies, including the Care Quality Commission (CQC) and Health and Safety Executive (HSE), did to address the identified poor care as well as asking questions of the local public engagement bodies and local coroner. The resulting Francis Report culminated in over 290 recommendations, which included that of revising stronger leadership in 'nursing and other professional values'.

Crucial to professional values is the nurse's self-awareness of their own moral and ethical values. Within the nurse-patient interaction, these values may often run up against the patient's own moral values and beliefs. Any such conflict may well weaken the patient's mental attitude and response to their illness. For example, religious and cultural differences have the potential to raise such conflicts, and 'a nurse-patient relationship that is fractured by a clash of ethical values, cultural insensitivity, disrespect and insults will not benefit the therapeutic relationship that every healthcare professional needs to foster' (Wheeler, 2012). However, during the course of the nurse's work, moral dilemmas which are often complex, may occur and cause interprofessional conflicts, for which the law may not always provide a solution. This could leave the nurse following their own notion of morals and whether their beliefs are ethically right. A hypothetical example may be that of a nurse caring for a patient with a painful terminal cancer, who, they believe, should be given a medical *Do Not Resuscitate* directive if the patient's condition worsens. However, the doctor may believe that the patient's life should be sustained and for treatment to be continued as per the religious principle of the sanctity of life. In this instance, neither the nurse or doctor are breaking the law; they are merely adhering to their own codes of professional conduct. Thus, their conflict is essentially of making a moral decision. Nevertheless, a number of such ethical dilemmas have been taken to the courts seeking a resolution to disagreements about the best way forward with the treatment and care of a particular patients. Therefore, such judgements by the courts are informed by moral analysis, and as Avery (2013) states, '…it is the lawyers who can frame the strongest moral argument that will win the day'.

In emphasising the necessity of professional values in reinforcing professional identity and practice, Elcock et al. (2019) stated, '…our practice as nurses must exemplify the integration of both the core standards of professional nursing and our inherent personal values in our clinical practice'. The Nursing and Midwifery Council (NMC), as the regulatory body for nurses, emphasises through its code for practice ('The Code') the proficiency standards for nurses through the public expectation that 'nurses possess the values and personal attributes of being caring, empathetic and compassionate' (NMC, 2018). Earlier policy work by the Chief Nursing Officer for England and the Chief Nursing Adviser for the Department of Health (DH) led to the formation of a set of core values for nursing, commonly known as the six 'Cs' (DH & NHS Commissioning Board, 2012): *care, compassion, communication, commitment, courage* and *competence*. These clearly emphasise practise driven by a values-led, patient-focussed mindset. For example, communication may have a span of varying verbal and non-verbal behaviour, but the underlying importance is of how the patient perceives the nurse as a caring professional. It is here that the nurse's personal values are required to interact with the expected core professional values.

There are various philosophical approaches to ethics, which constitute too large a subject matter to be explored within this text. Therefore, in Chapter 4, a description of a particular principles-based approach to ethical decision-making is made and applied to nursing.

References

Avery, G, 2013. Law and ethics in nursing and healthcare: an introduction. Sage Publications, London.

Beauchamp, TL, Childress, F, 2013. Principles of biomedical ethics, 7th ed. Oxford University Press, Oxford.

Brazier, M, Cave, E, 2016. Medicine, patients and the law, 6th ed. Penguin, London.

Department of Health, NHS Commissioning Board, 2012. Compassion in practice: nursing, midwifery and care staff – our vision and strategy. Available at: http://www.England.nhs.uk/wp-content/uploads/2012/12/compassion-in-practice.pdf.

Elcock, K, Wright, W, Newcombe, P, Everett, F, 2019. Essentials of nursing adults. Sage, London.

Francis, R, 2013. Report of the Mid Staffordshire Foundation Trust Public Inquiry. Executive Summary. The Stationery Office. Available at: https://assets.publishing.service.gov.uk.

Geldart, W, 1996. Introduction to English law, 11th ed. Oxford University Press, Oxford.

Herring, J, 2020. Medical law and ethics, 8th ed. Oxford University Press, Oxford.

Holmes, D, 2013. World report: Mid Staffordshire Scandal highlights NHS cultural crisis. The Lancet 381 (9866), 521–522.

National Health Service, 2013. The NHS Constitution for England. Available at: https://www.gov.uk/government/publications/the-nhs-constitution-for-england/the-nhs-constitution-for-england.

Nursing and Midwifery Council, 2018. The Code: professional standards of practice and behaviour for nurses, midwives and nursing associates. Available at: https://www.nmc.org.uk/standards/code/.

Oxford Dictionaries, 2011. Concise Oxford English dictionary, 12th ed. Oxford University Press, Oxford.

Oxford Dictionaries, 2018. Oxford dictionary of law, 9th ed. Oxford University Press, Oxford.

Seedhouse, D, 1998. Ethics: the heart of healthcare, 2nd ed. Wiley, Chichester.

Somerville, A, 2003. Judging law, ethics and intuition: practical answers to awkward questions. Journal of Medical Ethics 29, 281–286.

Thompson, M, 2019. Ethical theory, 4th ed. Hodder Education, London.

Wheeler, H, 2012. Law, ethics and professional issues in nursing: a reflective and portfolio-building approach. Routledge, London.

CASES

Bolam v Friern Hospital Management Committee [1957] 2 All ER 11
Donoghue v Stevenson [1932] AC 562
Chester v Afshar [2004] UKHL 41
R v Adomako [1995] 1 AC 171

STATUTES

Health and Safety at Work Act 1974
Equality Act 2010
National Health Service and Community Care Act 1990
Data Protection Act 1998

CHAPTER *2*

The Structure and Function of the Courts

KEY TERMS

UK courts

European Union legislation

Human Rights Act

Introduction

Through tradition and historical legislative development, there exists three distinct legal systems within the United Kingdom (UK), one each for England and Wales, Scotland and Northern Ireland. Since 1999, devolution has afforded the transfer of powers from Parliament in Westminster to the Welsh assembly in Cardiff, the Northern Irish Assembly in Belfast and the Scottish Parliament in Edinburgh. The Supreme Court of the United Kingdom has had jurisdiction over the entire UK since 2009, when it replaced the Judicial Committee of the House of Lords. These devolved assemblies derive their law-making authority from powers granted by the Parliament in Westminster. This textbook deals principally with the judicial processes of England and Wales, and where required makes relevant reference to the authority and influence of the European Union and the Human Rights Act 1998.

Figure 2.1 presents a diagram giving a structural overview of the UK Courts, with a description of the different courts and the influence of the European Courts.

The *Supreme Court* is the final court of appeal in the UK, and was established in 2009 to achieve a complete separation between the UK's senior judges and the Upper House of Parliament. This was to emphasise the independence of the Law Lords and increase the transparency between Parliament and the Courts, and the Law Lords who carried out the judicial work of the House of Lords left Parliament

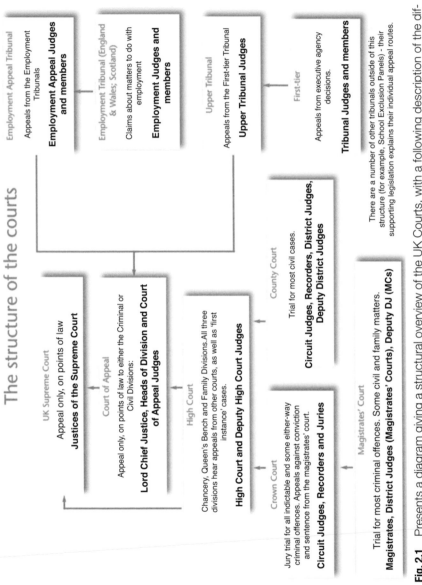

The structure of the courts

UK Supreme Court
Appeal only, on points of law
Justices of the Supreme Court

Court of Appeal
Appeal only, on points of law to either the Criminal or Civil Divisions:
Lord Chief Justice, Heads of Division and Court of Appeal Judges

High Court
Chancery, Queen's Bench and Family Divisions. All three divisions hear appeals from other courts, as well as 'first instance' cases.
High Court and Deputy High Court Judges

Crown Court
Jury trial for all indictable and some either-way criminal offences. Appeals against conviction and sentence from the magistrates' court.
Circuit Judges, Recorders and Juries

Magistrates' Court
Trial for most criminal offences. Some civil and family matters.
Magistrates, District Judges (Magistrates' Courts), Deputy DJ (MCs)

County Court
Trial for most civil cases.
Circuit Judges, Recorders, District Judges, Deputy District Judges

Employment Appeal Tribunal
Appeals from the Employment Tribunals
Employment Appeal Judges and members

Employment Tribunal (England & Wales; Scotland)
Claims about matters to do with employment
Employment Judges and members

Upper Tribunal
Appeals from the First-tier Tribunal
Upper Tribunal Judges

First-tier
Appeals from executive agency decisions.
Tribunal Judges and members

There are a number of other tribunals outside of this structure (for example, School Exclusion Panels) - their supporting legislation explains their individual appeal routes.

Fig. 2.1 Presents a diagram giving a structural overview of the UK Courts, with a following description of the different courts and the influence of the European Courts. Reproduced from https://www.judiciary.uk/wp-content/uploads/2016/05/international-visitors-guide-10a.pdf.

to become Justices of the new United Kingdom Supreme Court. This Court hears appeals on arguable points of law of the greatest public importance for civil cases in the UK. However, the Supreme Court must give effect to directly applicable EU law and interpret domestic law in a way that is consistent as far as possible. It also works under the influence of the rights contained in the European Convention of Human Rights and takes account of any decision of the European Court of Human Rights (ECtHR) in Strasbourg. The Supreme Court must also refer to the Court of Justice of the European Union (CJEU) and question EU law where the answer is not clear and is necessary for it to give judgement. Decisions are made, by unanimity or a simple majority, by the 12 appointed justices, and such decisions made in the Supreme Court or Court of Appeal become a precedent that must be followed by courts in all future cases.

The *High Court* comprises three divisions – the *Queen's Bench*, the *Chancery* and *Family*. Binding on lower court functions and usually involving one judge sitting alone, each has the authority to act as a court for hearing a case for the first time as well as being an appellate court. The Queen's Bench Division governs matters arising from cases that a Magistrates' Court may not be able to resolve as a point of law, and then it may ask the Divisional Court of the Queen's Bench to resolve such a matter. Thus, an appeal lies with the Divisional Court from the (lower) Crown Court where it has received an appeal from the Magistrates' Court. The prosecution or defence can further appeal through the Divisional Court to the Court of Appeal on a point of law, and as a first instance, the High Court (Queen's Bench) will hear particular medical and nursing negligence claims as major civil disputes. It is the Queen's Bench Division that administers common law relating to civil cases, and some of these cases from the High Court can jump ahead to be dealt with by the Supreme Court. The Chancery Division handles 'natural justice' cases mainly concerning equity, e.g. settling disputes concerning Wills and Trusts and those which concern matters of finance and property. The Family Division handles matters of family law, which include matrimonial disputes, adoption and the care of children, which may include medical treatment that is being contested. It also hears appeals from the Magistrates' Courts, county courts and the Crown Court.

The *Crown Court* sits in centres throughout England and Wales addressing indictable criminal cases that are transferred from the Magistrates' Courts. These are the more serious cases, which include murder, rape, manslaughter and robbery, and even though some defendants may be convicted in a Magistrates' Court, they may be transferred to the Crown Court for sentencing. The Crown Court also hears appeals against the decisions made by the magistrates. Cases are heard by a jury and a judge and the jury's decision will often be unanimous, although a judge may decide to accept a majority decision if it is found to be difficult for all 12 jurors to agree. During a trial, the judge advises the jury upon the law as well as being the person to impose a sentence upon any defendant proved to be 'guilty'. In criminal trials, appeals from the Crown Court lie with the Court of Appeals (Criminal Division), and such an appeal may be on a point of law or of fact, or against the sentence imposed. Only the defendant can appeal, and a successful appeal against a conviction can lead to the conviction being nullified or the magistrate court's decision being overturned. The Crown Court can also replace a conviction for some other offence for which the jury could have reached a decision for conviction.

Around 95% of all criminal cases are completed within the *Magistrates' Court*, and almost all criminal cases are heard by the Magistrates' Court on the first occurrence (Courts and Tribunals Judiciary, 2020). Serious cases may be reassigned to the Crown Court after an initial hearing by the magistrates; less serious cases and those involving juveniles are tried in the Magistrates' Courts. Some civil cases (e.g. matrimonial matters; adoption; child guardianship) are dealt with by the magistrates; however, these may be appealed to the County Courts. Cases are heard by three magistrates or by one district judge. In short, the Magistrates' Courts deal with less serious ('Summary Offence') cases. By contrast, cases which can be heard by the magistrates or before the judge and jury in a Crown Court ('Either-Way') or serious cases, such as murder, rape, manslaughter and robbery, which have to be tried in the Crown Court ('Indictable Only'). If a criminal offers a guilty plea to a summary offence, the magistrates give a sentence. If a not guilty plea is offered, then the case goes to trial. For a criminal found *guilty*, the Magistrates can then impose a sentence of up to 6 months imprisonment for a single offence and 12 months in total, or a fine of an unlimited sum. However, if a defendant is found *not guilty* of the criminal offence they were accused of, the defendant is deemed 'acquitted' and innocent in the eyes of the law and thus, free to go.

The *County Court* is a civil court concerned with cases of non-criminal and non-family matters where an individual or business believes their rights have been breached. These include a business trying to recover money or property (land) they are owed or a person(s) seeking compensation for injuries, for example, a workplace accident. It also assesses damages in uncontested cases and repossessions to recover losses. Those cases which involve large amounts of money, and those which are particularly complex, would be referred to the High Court to be dealt with. Most of these civil cases do not have a jury and the judge reads the case papers prior before hearing the case on his/her own. The judge manages the case throughout and controls its progress to expedite matters and for the parties involved to reach a settlement. After hearing evidence from all parties, the judge delivers their judgement and decides upon the amount of damages in the form of a monetary payment and the fees paid out by the parties, e.g. lawyers and court fees, expert witness contribution.

The Courts and Crime Act 2013 signalled the introduction of the *Family Court* in 2014. It brought all levels of the family judiciary to sit together in the same court with the benefit that time and resources were not lost in transferring cases between different courts as in the previous configuration. The Family Court comes under the judicial leadership of Designated Family Judges (DFJs) based within a designated centre in a particular geographical catchment area. Proceedings dispensed by the Family Court are given scrutiny by a legal adviser and district judge who allocate cases to the correct level of judge according to their type and complexity. Essentially there are two types of law case – private and public. The public cases are brought by local authorities or the NSPCC on matters such as Care Orders, Supervision

Orders or Emergency Protection Orders. Private cases generally are brought by persons on matters concerning divorce or parental separation e.g. custody of a child.

Coroner's Courts hold inquests into persons who have died suddenly, unnaturally, and/or as a result of an accident. At an inquest, the coroner will often sit alone but may summon a jury in particular cases, such as a death occurring in police custody or prison or under suspicious circumstances. A coroner can order a post mortem to establish the cause of death as part of the enquiry, and essentially an inquest is opened as a fact-finding process to establish the cause and circumstances surrounding a death. Integral to this process is that of ensuring the deceased is identified, that the death is officially recorded and that the body can be released for burial or cremation. Coroners are usually solicitors, barristers or medical practitioners of at least five years' experience, and they usually continue in their respective professional roles when not sitting in court. They were established in the year 1194, but the more recent Coroner and Justice Act 2009 created new laws and rules including the office of Chief Coroner, who assumes overall responsibility and leadership for coroners in England and Wales. Each locality has different levels of administration (including staffing) who are usually employed by the Local Authority and Police Authority for that locality.

A nurse, during their course of duties, may be involved in preparing a report upon events leading to the death of a patient and their involvement in the treatment and care of such. The nurse may be summoned to give evidence at a coroner's inquest, and the nurse has a duty to do so under the NMC Code of Practice (2015). Whereas for the nurse, this may feel rather daunting, the Coroners' Office exists to assist those called to attend the court; it is aware that persons giving evidence may be anxious and unsure about the pre-inquest processes. Published guidance for those attending the court has been made available (Ministry of Justice, 2020).

The Role of Religion

Since the 14th century, there has been an established legislative role of the church within Parliament by the existence of the Lords Spiritual. Today, 26 Church of England bishops form the Lords Spiritual with the existence of another 21 diocesan members, also serving in the House of Lords, and this religious influence has a continued presence within modern legislature. This religious presence has been the subject of critical debate, not more so than from the 'humanist' movement. Herring (2018) raises the point that religion can offer a 'challenging alternative' to orthodox approaches of medical ethics, but that many religious arguments are 'based on precepts which may not be readily open to challenge and negotiation'. However, some themes do appear to have a unified presence throughout different religions, for example, the 'sanctity of life'. An earlier opinion by Wickes (2009) emphasises that religion is an important part of decision-making concerning law, but it should not take priority over other moral considerations, with legislators needing to respect decisions that are for the whole of society, including those who take radically different views on religion and its role in private decisions amongst individuals within society.

The Influence of European Legislation

An increasing influence of law sources stems from 1973 with the UK's membership in the European Communities. Following the European Communities Act 1972, Article 249 EC said that regulation was to have a 'general application' and 'binding in every respect and directly applicable in all (EC) member states'. Directives resulting from such regulation inform the European Member States what needs to be done, but leave the Member States' governments to decide what requirements of national law are needed to enact and implement a directive.

Since 1966, UK citizens have had the right to petition the ECtHR, and developing from this, the Human Rights Act (1998) came into force in the year 2000, which allowed persons to rely directly in national courts on the rights guaranteed by the ECtHR. Based in Strasbourg, the ECtHR was established to address matters under the Human Rights Act, and cases could be launched as an appeal and go directly to the ECtHR, which establishes a number of fundamental rights and freedoms. Essentially, it has a regulatory, directive, and decision-making function in respect of addressing European case law, and it is the final avenue of complaint for individual citizens who have expended available national resolutions for alleged breaches of rights set out by the *European Convention of Human Rights* (the 'convention' formerly named the European Convention of Human Rights and Freedoms). The convention was founded by the Council of Europe in part due to the 1948 United Nations Declaration of Human Rights, and the Council of Europe was established in 1949 to secure international cooperation in preventing the atrocities of human rights which had taken place during the Second World War. The European Convention of Human Rights followed in 1950 and came into force in 1953, including endorsement by the UK, and established 14 fundamental rights and freedoms (Box 2.1).

The role of the *European Court of Justice (ECJ)*, also known as *the European Court of Justice of the European Union*, is to adjudicate between the EU and member states and upon disputes within the European community, e.g. a member state which fails to fulfil an EU directive. Based in Luxembourg, the ECJ consists of one judge from each EU member state and nine Advocates-General. National courts may make interim references directly to the ECJ if they need clarification on how a particular piece of EU legislation should be interpreted. Therefore, in England and Wales, the need for such references would occur in the Supreme Court, so if a court cannot make a ruling because it is unsure how to interpret a piece of EU legislation, then it may suspend the case before it in order to ask the ECJ for its judgement, referred to as an Article 234 reference. The case will then proceed in a UK court assisted by the ECJ ruling, and thus the role of the courts is to give effect to and enforce the rulings of the ECJ. Conversely, failure to comply with EU law may result in financial penalties imposed by the ECJ if a remedy is not found and the country is at fault, and the ECJ may also review the legality of a failure to act on the part of a community where the failure to act is deemed unlawful. It is the task of the institution of that country to take appropriate measures and put an end to the failure. Another function of the

---

BOX 2.1 ■ Convention Rights by Article Number

Article
1. Obligation to respect human rights
2. Right to life
3. Prohibition of torture
4. Prohibition of slavery and forced labour
5. Right to liberty and security
6. Right to a fair trial
7. No punishment without law
8. Right to respect for private and family life
9. Freedom of thought, conscience and religion
10. Freedom of expression
11. Freedom of assembly and association
12. Right to marry and found a family
13. Right to an effective remedy
14. Prohibition of discrimination

ECJ is to consider requests to withdraw (annul) a treaty or fundamental rights if an EU act is believed to infringe such by an EU Member State government. Individual persons may also ask the ECJ to withdraw an act that directly concerns them in some adverse way.

Human Rights Act 1998

The Human Rights Act (HRA) gives weight to the convention rights by requiring the UK courts to interpret the law in a manner that is compatible with this statute. Although the HRA does not directly incorporate the Human Rights Convention, the HRA initially requires that primary and delegated legislation be interpreted where possible in a manner which is compatible with convention rights. Thus, it is 'unlawful for a public authority to act in a way which is incompatible with a human right' (HRA, Sections 6–8). In UK law, judges endeavour to ensure that the common law is consistent with such Convention rights. Therefore, a judge hearing a medical claim from a person (e.g. patient) must consider compatibility with the Convention rights and ensure consistency in adhering to the Convention rights.

The most pertinent aspects of the HRA affecting the nurse and patient care are Articles 2, 3, 5, 8 and 14, briefly described as follows:

Article 2 states 'Everyone's *right to life* shall be protected by law. No one shall be deprived of his life intentionally save in the execution of a sentence of court following his conviction of a crime for which the penalty is provided by law'. Article 2 has raised a number of ethical dilemmas over the years, such as: Is it unlawful to withdraw treatment or feeding in cases of Persistent Vegetative State? or, does a viable foetus have a right to life? Matters concerning serious neglect or mistreatment would also be under the authority of this article. An example of the ethical and legal debate influenced by the HRA is that of *R v Swindon NHS PC Trust*, in which a woman was refused a potentially life-saving (but financially costly) breast cancer drug. The point was raised that Article 2 imposed on the state a positive obligation to intervene to protect people whose lives are at real and immediate risk, as raised in *Osman v UK*, and it was deemed that a patient whose life was endangered by refusal of a treatment could obtain a Court Order that they be given priority in treatment due to a breach of Article 2. The case of *Osman* also raised the matter that individual countries were allowed considerable freedom to assess their own aims and priorities even though the ECtHR has established well-defined provisions regarding the protection of persons from harm or disease requiring the use of state resources. Article 2 could apply to a normally competent person demanding an entitlement for the continuation of basic life-saving treatment as in the eminent case of *Burke* (Case Study 2.1).

Despite furthering his appeal to the European Court of Human Rights, Mr Burke lost his case (Burke v UK Application 19807/06).

The case of *Burke* presented a number of medico-ethical issues which divided opinion, such as a power shift from the medical professionals as decision-makers into the more autonomous hands of the patient as well as the courts. Also, the notion of 'best interests' occasioned much debate within the courts as to whether an objective test (a balance sheet of 'pros' and 'cons') was helpful when considering the rights of the incompetent patient, but also that a competent patient equating what was deemed their 'best interests' with their expressed wishes was unhelpful.

Article 3 provides that 'No one shall be subjected to torture or to inhuman or degrading treatment or punishment'. This could be used to challenge serious mistreatment, very poor care, or neglect. It may also concern a patient being restrained or secluded for aggressive behaviour, or a patient not being assisted to take food or fluids when too weak to do so themselves. The ethical arguments surrounding the legal prohibition of voluntary euthanasia could also be raised as being contrary to Article 3. For example, a person dying of an incurable, degenerative and perhaps

---

CASE STUDY 2.1	Burke v General Medical Council [2005] EWCA Civ 1003

Oliver Burke, a 45-year-old man suffering a congenital degenerative brain condition, challenged the General Medical Council (GMC) guidelines (*withdrawal of treatment for persistent vegetative state*) as an infringement of his human rights under Articles 2, 3 and 8. He demanded an entitlement for the continuation of artificial nutrition and hydration (ANH) as basic life-saving treatment even though his condition would deteriorate. The High Court ruled in his favour, implying that a competent person wishing to remain alive is legally entitled to receive life-sustaining treatment and that the doctors were obliged to continue with active treatment, even though some viewed it as futile, being that Mr Burke was considered to be in the terminal stages of life. However, through the Court of Appeal, the GMC successfully appealed against this judgement with the Court, insisting that a patient did not have a right to demand whatever treatment they wanted and that the duty to provide ANH was not an absolute duty and would also not apply if the patient was incompetent at some time in the future; in Mr Burke's situation, he may no longer be competent due to deteriorating health.

painful disease was denied the option of active euthanasia in that they were being subjected to inhuman and degrading treatment as emphasised in the case of *Pretty v UK*, which is given more detailed attention in Chapter 10 upon the law concerning death and dying. Article 5 provides that:

> Everyone has the right to liberty and security of person. No one shall be deprived of his liberty save the following cases* and in accordance with a procedure prescribed by law.

> *The lawful detention of persons for the prevention of the spreading of infectious diseases, of persons of unsound mind, and of alcoholics, drug addicts or vagrants; n.b. this would include mental health legislation.*

Depriving a person's liberty would include false imprisonment or being restrained to a bed or chair for long periods of time. However, under Section 47 of the National Assistance Act 1948 there is a power for the court to remove to a place of safety a person who is no longer able to care for themselves. In addition, Section 45G of the Public Health (Control of Disease) Act 1984, as amended by the Health and Social Care Act 2008, gives extensive powers to detain and treat patients who are infectious or contaminated and pose a risk to others.

Case Study 2.2 illustrates a UK 'landmark' case known as the 'Bournewood Judgement' which gives some explanation of the use of Article 5 within the judicial decision-making process. In this example the doctrine of necessity is defined as '...action to protect life or property in an emergency not caused by the defendant's negligence. The steps taken in the emergency must be reasonable' (Oxford Dictionaries, 2018).

CASE STUDY 2.2	**R v Bournewood Community Mental Health NHS Trust ex pL [1998] 1 AC 458**

This case involves a 49-year-old man (Mr L) with autism who, it was agreed, lacked capacity. In 1997 he was admitted to Bournewood Hospital and remained as an in-patient for almost 3 months. He was not detained under the Mental Health Act (MHA) 1983, but was accommodated for his own 'best interests' under the common law doctrine of 'necessity' despite his carers request for his discharge. Mr L's carers brought legal proceedings against the managers of the hospital, but the High Court rejected the claim and held that he had been detained in his lawful best interests under the common law doctrine of 'necessity'. Nevertheless, the Court of Appeal disagreed, taking the view that Mr L had been detained, and that such detention would only have been lawful under the MHA. Conversely, in agreeing with the High Court, the House of Lords reversed this decision.

Principally, the ECtHR agreed with the Court of Appeal, finding that Mr L was detained and that the 'right to liberty' in Article 5 of the Convention rights could be engaged and that detention under the Common Law was incompatible with Article 5 because it was too arbitrary and lacked sufficient safeguards, such as those available to patients detained under the MHA. Thus, the ECtHR held that judicial review was the only way Mr L had been able to challenge his common law detention, but this did not provide the rigorous challenge that was called for by the Convention's Article 5(4).

Bournewood was a significant case in that it pertained to the considerable numbers of people admitted to hospital under common law – in their 'best interests', and, as Diesfield (2000) noted, 'the concept of equality has been employed as a powerful ethical and legal instrument' in respect of the equal protection of people admitted to hospital.

Article 8 provides that 'Everyone has the right to respect for his private and family life, his home and his correspondence', and the obligations under Article 8 can appear more complex than other articles. For example, does it impose a duty not to interfere with a person's privacy or a positive obligation of the state to act to promote a right to privacy? Article 8, for example, could include a person wanting more privacy in a residential home; not wanting to be in a mixed-sex hospital ward; wanting to discuss a medical problem in private; or their spiritual and family needs not been met whilst in care. There are exceptions to the statement of provision under Article 8(2), which stipulates that it could be infringed '...in the interests of national security, public safety or the economic well-being of the country, for the prevention of disorder or crime, for the protection of health or morals, or for the protection of the rights and freedoms of others'.

The high-profile media case (Case Study 2.3) of *Campbell v MGN* illustrates how HRA Articles can give different perspectives, and in some instances, conflicting perspectives on a legal case.

The *Campbell* decision emphasised a robust and persuasive privacy right to 'protect' despite there being a public interest in publishing particular information. This high level of protection under Article 8 could be attained by the proportionality exercise of the case, which, if tested, raises the questions of whether there was a

---

CASE STUDY 2.3   **Campbell v MGN [2004] UKHL 22**

Supermodel Naomi Campbell (named 'C') had publicly denied that she took illicit drugs, but the Mirror Group Newspapers (MGN) published editorials regarding her alleged addiction, including showing photographs of her leaving a Narcotics Anonymous group therapy meeting. C sought damages for a breach of her confidentiality relating to the surreptitious photographs, but accepted that the newspaper was entitled to publish that she had a drug addiction and was receiving treatment, thus rescinding her previous denial of such. C was successful at trial, following consideration under Article 8, of which it was held that the information complained of was confidential and that publication of such was not in the public interest. However, the Court of Appeal allowed the newspaper's appeal on the basis that the new information (C's addiction treatment) was in the public interest under Article 10 ('freedom of expression') and necessary for the journalistic plausibility of the story.

C appealed to the House of Lords, who upheld her appeal in that her therapy as a recovering addict rendered her health vulnerable, both physically and mentally, and that the details of her therapy constituted private information giving rise to a duty of confidentiality. In this instance, there was little public interest and the freedom of the press journalists had exceeded the public interest; the photographs had infringed a reasonable expectation of privacy and were likely to cause C distress. This case could be viewed as having a result whereby 'the right to privacy trumped the right to freedom of expression' (Herring, 2020).

reasonable expectation of privacy at stake, and whether the privacy claim was stronger than the free speech claim.

Article 14 requires that all of the HRAs rights and freedoms must be protected and applied without discrimination. Discrimination is defined as 'treating a person less favourably than others on grounds unrelated to merit, usually because he or she belongs to a particular group or category' (Oxford Dictionaries, 2018). Therefore, it is unlawful to discriminate on grounds of race, sex (including gender reassignment), sexual orientation, religion or belief, disability or age. The Equality and Human Rights Commission (2018) emphasised that to rely on Article 14, 'you must show that discrimination has affected your enjoyment of one or more of the other rights of the Act, even though you do not need to prove that this other right has been breached'.

The Equality Act (2010), which offers more general protection, came into force by bringing together into one single Act nine main pieces of legislation, which included the Sex Discrimination Act 1975; the Race Relations Act 1976; and the Disability Discrimination Act 1995. This Act provided a legal framework to protect the rights of individuals and advance equal opportunity for all in the UK, and exists to protect individuals from unfair treatment and promote a fair and more equal society (Equality and Human Rights Commission, 2019).

It is essential for the nurse to grasp the essence of Article 14 (non-discrimination) within their practice. This requires a credible level of self-awareness in terms of values, beliefs and understanding of others with whom they communicate, who may be from a different cultural background with different experiences and presenting differing viewpoints and beliefs. These differences may include those of ethnicity, religion, gender, sexuality and disability. As such, conflicts or dilemmas may arise for the nurse, who may have their own pre-conceived perspectives about certain types of people, but who would be aided by gaining further insight into the broader society. Such developed insight would benefit the nurse when practising in a non-discriminatory way which is mindful of individual and cultural differences of the people they care for and work alongside. Such insight serves to demonstrate a more principled respect and understanding of patients, their relatives and carers, as well as other professionals. These principles extend throughout the law and ethics concerning medicine and nursing, and with a grasp of the fundamental premise of the Human Rights Act, such principles help provide a sound, safe and competent foundation for the professional nurse working within the bounds of domestic and European law.

References

Courts and Tribunals Judiciary, 2020. You and the Judiciary. Available at: www.judiciary.uk.

Diesfield, D, 2000. Neither consenting nor protecting: an ethical analysis of a man with autism. Journal of Medical Ethics 26, 277–281.

Equality and Human Rights Commission, 2018. Human Rights Act. Available at: https://www.equalityhumanrights.com/en/human-rights-act/article-14-protection-discrimination.

Equality and Human Rights Commission, 2019. Available at: https://www.equalityhuman-rights.com/en.

Herring, J, 2020. Medical law and ethics, 8th ed. Oxford University Press, Oxford.

Ministry of Justice, 2020. Guide to coroner services. Available at: https://www.gov.uk/government/publications/guidetocoronersservices.

Nursing and Midwifery Council, 2015. The Code: professional standards of practice and behaviour for nurses, midwives and nursing associates. Available at: https://www.nmc.org.uk/standards/code.

Oxford Dictionaries, 2018. Oxford dictionary of law, 9th ed. Oxford University Press, Oxford.

Wicks, E, 2009. Religion, law and medicine: legislating on birth and death in a Christian state. Medical Law Review 17 (3), 410–437.

CASES

Burke v General Medical Council [2005] EWCA Civ 1003
Burke v UK Application 19807/06 (2006)
Campbell v MGN [2004] UKHL 22
Osman v UK (1998) 29 EHRR 245
Pretty v United Kingdom [2002] 2 FLR 45
R v Swindon NHS PC Trust [2006] EWCA Civ 392
R v Bournewood Community Mental Health NHS Trust ex pL [1998] 1 AC 458

STATUTES

Coroner and Justice Act 2009
Courts and Crime Act 2013
Disability Discrimination Act 1995
European Communities Act 1972
Health and Social Care Act 2008
Human Rights Act 1998
National Assistance Act 1948
Race Relations Act 1976
Sex Discrimination Act 1975

The Professional Nurse and the Law

KEY TERMS

Accountability
Standard of care
Fitness to practice

Duty of candour
Serious incidents

Introduction

The term *professional* is frequently used to describe the role, expectations and activity of a particular type of worker. However, how often does the nurse consider what the term means to them? Of equal importance is the significance of being a professional nurse and the legislation that regulates the actions of a person deemed to be a professional nurse. Oxford Dictionary defines 'profession' as 'having or showing the skill of a professional, competent... engaged in a specific activity as one's own main paid occupation... a vocation or calling... one that involves some kind of advanced learning or science' (Concise Oxford Dictionary, 2011). Professional skills define the specific activities that a nurse (or other professionals) needs to learn and perform, and the abilities (which may vary in complexity) to perform specific activities required of the nursing role. For example, an A&E nurse may well have skills different from a mental health nurse; however, it is reasonable to assume that both possess the fundamental skill of communicating with people. This combination of knowledge, skills and ability helps a nurse reach a certain level of competence required for their role. It is when the nurse's performance of their duties falls below the expected level of competence that matters arise, which need to be addressed and acted upon through the processes of regulatory law.

Professional Accountability

Accountability is a term that has various meanings and implications. Being 'accountable' can have simple definitions, such as 'required to account for one's conduct' (Concise Oxford Dictionary, 2011); 'accepting ownership for the results' (Sullivan and Garland, 2010) or 'explain and justify actions or non-actions' for a given responsibility (Barr and Dowding, 2016). By contrast, within the professional context, accountability broadens to specific areas of the nurse's role. Based on the belief that there is no single source of accountability for nurses and that different authorities create different structures and standards, Caulfield (2005) addressed this issue by devising a framework of accountability that considers the varying standards and types of authority. This framework consists of four key types of accountability: professional, ethical, legal, and employment (see Fig. 3.1). As previously mentioned, there are different authorities who exercise standards and specify expected behaviours from nurses. Thus, accountability covers a broad spectrum of nurses' professional conduct. For example, if a nurse is found to have stolen money and/or valuables from a patient, the employer may instigate some disciplinary action as well as report the matter to the police and the nursing regulator. Aside from action from such bodies of authority, the nurse and their employing organisation have a duty to be open, honest and transparent with the affected patient; this is known as the *duty of candour*.

Professional accountability is exercised by the government that establishes regulation as a form of state control on behaviour, the healthcare provider environment

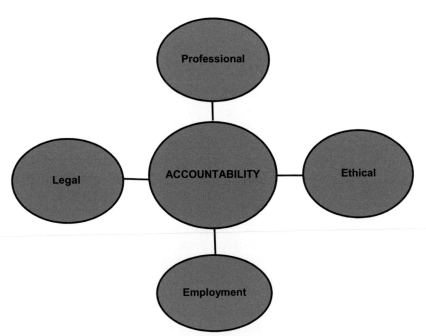

Fig 3.1 A framework of accountability. (Based on Caulfield, 2005.)

and the quality of the care in that environment. It establishes a framework of practice and principles of conduct expected of a nurse, and a personal relationship of the nurse with the body of regulation that sets standards and limits on professional accountability – currently the Nursing and Midwifery Council (NMC). Fundamental to such accountability is the moral belief of nursing being predicated on promoting the safety and welfare of patients in their care and on following the principles of conduct that promote trust in the nurse by the patient and the society at large, through their perspective of the profession. The NMC decides the prerequisites for a person to enter the nursing profession and sets the conditions for a person to be removed; it maintains a code of conduct, outlining minimum standards of behaviour expected of professional nurses and midwives.

Ethical accountability implies that a nurse will have their own moral values, and in recognising such, are aware when their own values are challenged by different values held by others. Ethics provides for much debate concerning moral values, even though it may not provide answers within the clinical context. Termination of pregnancy is an example that arouses much debate, primarily due to a conflict of moral values held by both clinicians and other individuals and spheres of society. Respect for the patient's right to choose what happens to their body and respect for their choice of lifestyle, contentment and personal dignity – in other words, the patient's autonomy – is a key ethical principle that nurses must consider. However, in situations where a person is unable to exercise their autonomy, then broader public policy deliberations may prioritise society's ethics over the rights of the individual patient. This can create conflict, leading to the civil courts enforcing law to ensure that matters progress in the best interests of the patient. Conversely, actions that disregard a competent patient's autonomy may be regarded as paternalistic. Indeed, for decades, healthcare providers have been criticised for adopting a paternalistic 'doctor knows best' approach to patient treatment and care, where there was an assumed understanding that the professional's advice and instructions were the accepted course of action. This conflict of values between autonomy and medical/nursing paternalism remains. Consequently, the nurse's self-awareness is essential to achieve the best balance between the patient's right to choose and what is considered best medical/nursing practice. An ethical framework is detailed further in Chapter 4.

A lack of understanding of nurses' *legal accountability* can lead to defensive nursing practices, where the potential risk of legal action is placed above the needs of the patient (Caulfield, 2005). Historically, a majority of health law cases in court focus on medical decisions and actions rather than nursing; nevertheless, it is essential for nurses to develop a working understanding of how the principles of law apply to their practice. Patients and carers are increasingly exercising their rights as service users by becoming better informed about their entitlements and legal rights. Indeed, litigation and financial compensation claims (e.g. in negligence cases) against healthcare providers have increased, as has media interest. However, it is important for the nurse to be aware that the law serves to not only protect the patient, but also to protect and guide the nurse as a professional in being able to validate and be accountable for their decisions in practice.

The employment contract is the foundation for the nurse's *employment account-ability*, which specifies a relationship with the employer and stipulates the duties and responsibilities that both parties agree to be accountable for. A job description is often provided, which further details the extent of the contracted duties, as well as the protocols and policies that lay down specific undertakings within the employer-employee relationship. This assists in ensuring that the nurse, under the Employment Rights Act 1996, has some recourse to a body, such as an employment tribunal, if they are treated unfairly, and that the employer has recourse (e.g. disciplinary pro-ceedings) if a nurse does not perform within the terms stipulated in the employ-ment contract. The health and safety of all workers, including nurses, is another important aspect of employment accountability. All workers have a responsibility to practise safely and report any accidents, hazards and potentially serious risks to their employer. Equally, the employer has the responsibility and duty to maintain a safe working environment for its employees under the Health and Safety at Work etc Act 1974 section 2(1), which states that 'it shall be the duty of every employer to ensure, as far as reasonably practicable, the health, safety, and welfare at work of all his employees'. This health and safety responsibility extends to acts or omissions upon patients and those who visit or use hospital or care provider premises under the doctrine of 'vicarious liability', which means that '…an employer is liable for the negligence of their employees who are acting in the course of their employment' (Herring, 2020). Even though the provider organisation may be held liable under law for any harm caused to a patient, the nurse should not assume that this pro-vides a shield from liability for their own independent decisions and practice. The repercussions for the nurse of an inquiry, inquest or court case may result in action taken through the employer's own disciplinary proceedings and through the legal processes of the NMC as the professional regulator.

Nursing and Midwifery Council – The Nursing Regulator

The NMC has been the regulator for nurses since the Parliament implemented the Nursing and Midwifery Order 2001, which brought nursing and midwifery practice under the control of statute and case law. The NMC is one of 15 healthcare regula-tors in the UK, which include the General Medical Council and General Dental Council. Accordingly, as with other regulators, the NMC is also under regulatory control by the Health Professions Council (HPC), an independent health regula-tor formed through statute by the Health Professions Order 2001. Throughout this textbook, the roles and functions of the NMC will be discussed with reference to nurses; however, these also apply to the midwives and nursing associates.

In protecting the wellbeing and safety of the public, the NMC has four key functions:

- Maintaining a register of nurses and midwives who meet the requirements for UK registration, and nursing associates who meet the requirements for registration in England.

- Setting the requirements of professional education that helps people develop knowledge, skills and behaviours required for entry to the register.
- Shaping the practice of the professionals on the register by developing and promoting standards, which include the Code of Practice (2018), and promoting lifelong learning through revalidation.
- Where serious concerns are raised about a registrant's fitness to practice, the NMC can investigate, and take action if required.

The Nursing and Midwifery Council's 'Code of professional standards of practice and behaviour' (NMC, 2018a), hereafter known as the *Code*, was developed in 2008 to serve as a framework for establishing standards for nurses and midwives in safeguarding the health and well-being of the public. Its primary focus is to ensure that nurses practise according to the code in providing high standards of care. The *Code* was revised in 2015 and more recently in 2018 to include nursing associates, who are now subject to the same regulations. In linking professionalism with the *Code*, Wheeler (2012) asserted that being a professional is the quality of '... being dedicated, committed, hard-working, competent, responsible and accountable for his/her professional actions and omissions too, and for his/her behaviour on the job and in private life too'. Even though the *Code* is validated, a nurse may well be faced with ethical dilemmas arising from a discord between personal and professional values; therefore, as a framework, it has been described as interpretative (Buka, 2015). The four main sections of the code are outlined in Box 3.1 (below).

Competence and the Standard of Care?

Implicit within the NMC Code is *practising care effectively and safely*. The NMC, through the Nursing and Midwifery Order (2001), is required to establish standards for education and training necessary for a nurse to achieve the required proficiency to be admitted to the register. To this end, the NMC has produced proficiency standards which are to be worked towards from the beginning of a nurse's undergraduate education to the completion following a programme of continuous assessment. The emphasis is on knowledge, skills and proficiency. Therefore, the newly registered nurse will embark on a pathway that is governed by policy (national and local), protocols and guidelines. The nurse's actual clinical practice will be overseen by the employing healthcare providers' organisational shared governance policy. Such a policy may work for differing protocols across clinical specialisms, with all nurses being subject to varying levels of scrutiny, management and supervision. However, there is no template for a nurse to practice at a high level of ability where they are completely free of the potential to make an error of judgment or lapse into incompetence. Although the qualified nurse is deemed an independent practitioner in their own right, their accountability extends to their teamworking competence and cooperation with other agencies to provide a safe, high standard of care to patients. Over the past 20 years, nurses have extended their professional knowledge and skills to roles of a higher responsibility that were previously only undertaken by medical practitioners. Consequently, the nurse's judgement and decision-making involves more complex moral, ethical and

BOX 3.1 ■ **The NMC Code of professional standards of practice and behaviour for nurses, midwives and nursing associates (2018)**

Prioritise people

- Treat people as individuals and uphold their dignity
- Listen to people and respond to their preferences and concerns
- Make sure that people's physical, social and psychological needs are assessed and responded to
- Act in the best interests of people at all times
- Respect people's rights to privacy and confidentiality

Practise effectively

- Always practise in line with the best available evidence
- Communicate clearly
- Work co-operatively
- Share your skills, knowledge and experience for the benefit of people receiving care and your colleagues
- Keep clear and accurate records relevant to your practice

Preserve safety

- Recognise and work within the limits of your competence
- Be open and candid with all service users about all aspects of care and treatment, including when any mistakes or harm have taken place
- Always offer help if an emergency arises in your practice setting or anywhere else
- Act without delay if you believe that there is a risk to patient safety or public protection
- Raise concerns immediately if you believe a person is vulnerable or at risk and needs extra support and protection
- Advise on prescribe, supply, dispense or administer medication within the limits of your training and competence, the law, our guidance and other relevant policies, guidance and regulations
- Be aware of, and reduce as far as possible, any potential for harm associated with your practice

Promote professionalism and trust

- Uphold the reputation of your profession at all times
- Uphold your position as a registered nurse, midwife or nursing associate
- Fulfil all registration requirements
- Cooperate with all investigations and audits
- Respond to any complaints made against you professionally
- Provide leadership to make sure people's wellbeing is protected and to improve their experiences of the health and care system

Adapted from *The Code* (2018a) Nursing and Midwifery Council

clinical dilemmas. Such dilemmas require nurses working in these extended roles to have a working knowledge of the law linked to professional responsibilities, particularly when their practice comes under some form of legal inquiry.

CASE STUDY 3.1	**Bolam v Friern Hospital Management Committee [1957] 1 WLR 583**

Mr Bolam (the claimant) agreed to undergo electroconvulsive therapy treatment (ECT) for a severe depressive illness. The anaesthetist did not administer a muscle relaxant drug and Mr Bolam fractured his hip bones due to violent convulsions. However, the opinion among medical practitioners about the effectiveness and risk of administering a muscle relaxant was divided. Mr Bolam sued the hospital for compensation, claiming a breach of duty by the doctor in not giving the muscle relaxant drug, failing to restrain him during the procedure and not warning him of the risks involved with ECT. His legal counsel also produced expert witnesses to assist his case.

However, the House of Lords Judge found that the doctor was not in breach of duty and ruled in favour of the hospital, stating, 'A medical professional is not guilty of negligence if he has acted in accordance with a practice accepted as proper by a responsible body of medical men skilled in that particular art…a man is not negligent, if he is acting in accordance with such a practice, merely because there is a body of opinion who would take a contrary view'.

The law governing the nurse's standard and duty of care falls under the canopy of medical case law concerning doctors and allied health professionals. To illustrate, the case of *Bolam v Friern Hospital Management Committee* (Case study 3.1) details a court judgement regarding what constitutes as acceptable, competent clinical practice despite a patient's claim of injury.

The reasoning behind what came to be known as the 'Bolam test' was rationalised in *Maynard v West Midlands RHA*, where it was held that a judge is not in a position to choose between the views of competing expert medical opinions. Thus, if there was a competent school of thinking that believed the doctor's (defendants) actions were reasonable, then the judge would not find the doctor negligent. *Sidaway v Board of Governors* also demonstrated the use of *Bolam* in judicial decision-making. More recently, the case of *Bolitho v City and Hackney Health Authority* narrowed the scope of the *Bolam* test. The *Bolitho* judgement stated that the court must be satisfied that the body of opinion relied upon has a logical basis and risks and benefits have been properly considered, emphasising that the judge must provide reasons for rejecting medical opinion and where expert evidence is given greater scrutiny.

Fitness to Practise

The (NMC, 2020a) defines 'fitness to practise' (FTP) as: 'being fit to practice requires a nurse, midwife or nursing associate to have the skills, knowledge, health and character to do their job safely and effectively'. In possessing the requirements to be fit to practise, the NMC had detailed a structure of standards of proficiency which 'represent the knowledge, skills and attributes that all registered nurses must demonstrate when caring for people of all ages and across all care settings… (and) reflect what the public can expect nurses to know and be able to do in order to deliver safe, compassionate and effective nursing care' (NMC, 2018b).

If there are concerns or complaints about a nurse's FTP safely, then a referral can be made to the NMC by an employer, a healthcare colleague, another healthcare regulator or a member of the public, including the Police. A formal legal process is then entered into and can take up to 15 months to complete; during this time, the referrals are considered and based upon particular key principles concerning allegations of fraudulent or incorrect entry into the register, misconduct, lack of competence, criminal convictions and cautions, health (affecting ability to practice safely), not having the necessary knowledge of the English language and determinations made by other referring healthcare organisations. The NMC has both nurse/midwife and lay members who work with the process of addressing such referrals; to judge FTP, they form a committee, which has the authority to impose sanctions upon a registrant on the grounds of either public safety and/or public interest.

The seriousness of concerns raised through such referrals are assessed by the NMC, who review the risks that are likely to arise if the nurse does not remedy or rectify the concerns. This is usually around potential harm to patients if not rectified and/or concerns based on the need to promote public confidence in nurses. Initially, an NMC case examiner considers all the information provided and decides whether there is a case to answer. If they decide that there is no case to answer, the matter may be closed, or they may decide to issue advice, a warning or recommend undertakings that must be agreed to by the registrant. However, when there is a case to answer and the matters are of serious concern, the case may be referred to a meeting or a hearing held by an FTP committee, which comprises a panel with both registrants and lay persons. Where the NMC is unable to decide upon a referral, the case examiner may refer to an Investigating Committee for a decision, which may still result in referral to the FTP Committee. The FTP committee panel then exercises its own judgement to decide whether the nurse's FTP is impaired, and the reasons for impairment; for example, whether the nurse's behaviour amounted to misconduct (NMC, 2020b). When making this decision, the panel considers the standards and behaviour expected of a registered nurse, midwife or nursing associate, who would be ordinarily working at the level of practice, but not necessarily at the highest possible level. Abiding by NMC guidance and referring to the *Code*, the panel, after considering the presented documentary evidence and witness testimony through cross-examination, will decide whether to impose one of the following sanctions:

- No further action/case to answer
- Issue a caution for a period of between 1 and 5 years
- Impose conditions of practice for a period of up to 3 years
- Suspend the registrant from the register for up to 1 year
- Strike the nurse off the register; they can re-apply for registration after a period of 5 years

Referrals to the NMC can be made if a nurse has a longstanding untreated health condition, an unsuccessfully treated health condition or a relapse of an existing condition which is cause for concern as it hampers the nurse's ability to practice safely. In such cases, the NMC may have to consider imposing some form of restriction upon the nurse to ensure that there is no risk of harm to patients or others (NMC, 2020b). When considering the ability to practise affected by health cases, as with cases concerning lack of competence or impairment due to a lack knowledge of English, the FTP committee cannot impose a striking-off order, if this is the first time the case is heard. This sanction can only be applied if the registrant has been continuously suspended or subject to a condition of practise order for the previous 2 years. Some or all aspects of a 'health' case can be heard in private to protect the anonymity of any alleged victims, or if any evidence shared is of a confidential medical nature. Hence, if a nurses' FTP is alleged to be impaired because of their health, then the hearing can be held in private (NMC, 2020b).

The demonstration of insight is a crucial factor for the panel. This may include the registrant's ability to 'step-back' and view the situation objectively, recognise what went wrong, appreciate what could and should have been done differently with the responsibilities assigned to them within their particular clinical role. Remediation is a significant factor for the FTP panel's deliberations (NMC, 2020b). After viewing the presented evidence and cross examination of the registrant and witnesses, the panel then decides upon whether the registrant's FTP is impaired and considers critical aspects such as the nurse's level of insight and whether the concerns about their practice are remediable. Matters concerning poor record keeping or medication administration errors may be viewed as examples that are easier to remedy than violent, abusive or neglectful behaviour towards patients and criminal convictions leading to a custodial sentence (NMC, 2020b). The NMC seeks evidence that the nurse has taken 'sufficient remedial steps' (NMC, 2020b), which may include attending training courses with some form of assessment; a critical written reflection with examples, reflecting whether the nurse has learned to address concerns made about their practice; or supervision records and testimonials from the nurse's employer with regard to observed good practice, behaviour and attitude which has addressed the concerns identified by the NMC FTP panel. The NMC's FTP has guidance on 'serious concerns which are more difficult to put right' (NMC, 2020b). It specifies that 'serious concerns' would include such acts as direct physical and sexual assault; giving a false picture of employment history; exploiting potential for financial gain; exposing patients to harm or neglect; deliberate causation of harm to patients and longstanding dishonesty within the nurse's clinical practice.

Remediation was emphasised by Dame Janet Smith in the Shipman Enquiry (The Shipman Enquiry Fifth Report, 2004), who recommended that a test be applied by healthcare regulator FTP panels to assist their decision-making as to whether a practitioner's conduct and performance was impaired. That is, have the concerns about practice been remedied or is it likely that the conduct will be repeated? This test was described in the case of *Council for Healthcare Regulatory Excellence v Nursing and Midwifery Council and another* (2011). The enquiry resulted from investigations into a General Practitioner (GP) who was a serial killer in England and given a life sentence, having been found guilty in January 2000 for murdering 15 of his patients by injecting them with diamorphine. In the subsequent sixth report of the enquiry, it was concluded that he had killed about 250 patients, mainly women, between 1971 and 1998. His motive was one of enjoying watching the process of dying and the sense of power and control he felt over a person's life. This case was an extreme example of a healthcare practitioner's contempt for both humanity and morality, as well as the ethical code required to treat and care for vulnerable persons. In the enquiry's fifth report, Dame Janet Smith, Chief of the Enquiry, made recommendations for improvements to patient complaints systems, methods of monitoring, managing and disciplining GPs, and for reforming the system of medical regulation and modifying the regulatory FTP functions. Although the enquiry focussed upon the practice of GPs, its recommendations were directed towards healthcare regulators in improving their processes of addressing patient safety through more effective regulation of clinical practitioner competence and accountability. In emphasising the implications of the enquiry, one critic stated that the General Medical Council as a regulator had 'tended to place the interests of doctors before the interests of patients' (Baker, 2005).

This chapter presents only a brief overview of the NMC's duties in regulating nursing and the process of decision-making and action through the FTP rules. For more comprehensive detail and guidance, as well as for essential reference purposes, the reader is advised to refer to the NMC website at https://www.nmc.org.uk.

Duty of Candour

Integral to the FTP requirements is the professional duty of candour, where there is a need to avoid breaches of such a duty and to 'be open and honest when things go wrong…', which includes '…covering up, falsifying records, obstructing, victimising or hindering a colleague or member of staff or patient who wants to raise a concern, encouraging others not to tell the truth or otherwise contributing to a culture which suppresses openness about the safety of care' (NMC, 2020b). Scrutiny of such concerns often gives rise to examination of any evidence of dishonest behaviour by a nurse. The court cases of *Parkinson v Nursing and Midwifery Council*, *R v Ghosh* and *Ivey v Ghenting Casinos* refer to judgements principally concerning dishonesty. Over the years, these cases have been referred to when making judgements relating specifically to the regulation of conduct of clinical practitioners. During the *Ghosh* case, the judge set a two-part test in establishing whether dishonesty was evident. The first (objective) test was whether 'according to the ordinary standards of reasonable and honest people', what was done by the defendant was dishonest. If it was not dishonest by those standards, then the second part (subjective) test was for the court (or panel) to consider whether the defendant (registrant) themselves must have known that what they were doing was, by those standards, dishonest. However, the more recent case of *Ivey* has provided a test which has superseded *Ghosh*. This is described in Case study 3.2, as follows:

Ivey overturned *Ghosh* in formulating a new test for the criminal and civil courts when determining the element of dishonesty in legal proceedings, and removed the requirement that 'the defendant must appreciate that what he has done is, by those

CASE STUDY 3.2	Ivey v Genting Casinos [2017] UKSC 67

Phil Ivey, a high-stakes professional (gambling) card player, brought a claim against Genting Casinos as they had refused to pay him his £7.7 million winnings, stating that he had cheated. Ivey used a technique concerning the card-deck called 'edge-scoring' and persuaded the croupier to rearrange the cards based upon Ivey's 'super-stitious' nature, which led to high value cards being placed in the 'shoe'. Even though both parties agreed that a betting contract implied that neither party would cheat, Ivey argued that 'cheating' required an element of dishonesty and that the casino had not established this. The Court of Appeal agreed with the original decision and found against Ivey, who then took the matter to the Supreme Court. In determining whether Ivey was cheating, the Supreme Court scrutinised the broader definition of dishonesty using a new test from that of *Ghosh*. It held that a court:

- First, 'must ascertain (subjectively) the actual state of the individual's knowledge or beliefs as to the facts. The reasonableness, or otherwise, of his belief may evidence whether he held the belief, but it is not an additional requirement that his belief must be reasonable; the question is whether it is genuinely held'.
- Second, once this (above) has been established, the court must determine 'whether his conduct was dishonest by applying the objective standards of ordinary decent people. It is not necessary for the individual to appreciate that what he has done is, by those standards, dishonest'.

Satisfied that the requirements of this test had been met, the Supreme Court dismissed Ivey's appeal.

standards, dishonest' – in effect, the defendant's own personal perception of dishonesty. In objecting to the second leg of *Ghosh*, the Supreme Court expressly stated that '...the principal objection is that the less a defendant's standards conform to society's expectations, the less likely they are to be held criminally responsible for their behaviour. The law should not excuse those who make a mistake about contemporary standards of honesty, a purpose of the criminal law is to set acceptable standards of behaviour' (Supreme Court, 2017). In effect, *Ghosh* brought dishonesty in line with other breaches of the law that operated under the principle of *mens rea* (Latin, meaning the intention to bring about a particular consequence).

The Health and Social Care Act 2008 (Regulated Activities) Regulations 2014: Regulation 20, states that Registered Persons must act in an open and transparent way with relevant persons in relation to care and treatment provided to service users in carrying out regulated activities. In Wales, the National Health Service (Concerns, complaints and redress arrangements) (Wales) Regulations 2011 made directives equivalent to those of Regulation 20 in England. Regulation 20 was introduced as a direct response to Recommendation 181 of the Francis Inquiry Report into the Mid-Staffordshire Foundation Trust (Francis, 2013). The inquiry report recommended that a statutory duty of candour be introduced for health and care providers and that this be a contractual requirement in the NHS and a professional requirement in the 'practise of regulated activity'; nursing would be an example of a regulated activity. Regulation 20 stipulates that 'as soon as reasonably practical' after being made aware that a notifiable safety incident has occurred, a registered person must notify the relevant person (e.g. patient) that the incident has occurred and 'provide reasonable support' to such a person in relation to the incident (Francis, 2013). This duty of candour applies to all organisations registered with the health-care regulator – the Care Quality Commission (CQC) in England. If a provider organisation, either NHS or independent, fails to comply with the duty of can-dour, it may be subject to action by the CQC, including criminal prosecution in serious cases. The CQC adheres to the Francis Report's duty of candour, linking it directly to the requirement of enabling concerns and complaints to be raised freely with questions to be answered, as well as openness which allows informa-tion regarding the truth about performance to be shared with staff, patients, the public and regulators – 'transparency' (CQC, 2015).

Organisational Meaning of a 'Serious Incident'

What then constitutes a 'serious incident'? While this may appear obvious, the spec-trum is now more far-reaching than before due to its evolution since 2000, the year that witnessed the kickstart of the patient safety movement in the UK follow-ing the publication of the report, 'An Organisation with a Memory' (Department of Health, 2000). This government report recommended the implementation of a new approach in responding to 'adverse events' (now known as 'patient safety incidents'), better systems-thinking, cultural change towards blame-free report-ing and learning from other high-risk industries, such as aviation. Building on these recommendations, the National Patient Safety Agency (NPSA) was created in 2001. This special health authority has devised and promoted national guidance for patient safety improvement, including a national reporting system of safety incidents for implementation throughout the NHS (NPSA, 2004). This National Reporting and Learning System (NRLS) provides consistent and detailed data regarding the occurrence and nature of safety incidents, which are open to public scrutiny and maintained within a managed database. The 'Seven Steps to Patient Safety' (2004) was the principal document outlining the developing work of the NPSA, until such safety policies were taken over by NHS Improvement in 2016. The document set a precedent for NHS Trusts to use its resources to develop their own patient safety protocols and practices, such as patient safety incident report-ing, investigation, root cause analysis and staff training, as well as being a prelude to a duty of candour with the document's acknowledgement of truthfulness and the 'principle of apology' (NPSA, 2004).

In continuing the formative work of the NPSA, NHS England (2015) set out further protocols and guidance to assist NHS providers. It defined a 'serious inci-dent' as 'acts/omissions that result in avoidable death, which includes suicide, homi-cide or serious self-harm; unexpected or avoidable injury to one or more people that requires further treatment by a healthcare professional in order to prevent death of such persons; serious harm or alleged abuse (sexual, physical or psychological) and acts of omission which constitute neglect, exploitation, financial or material abuse' (NHS England, 2015). Also included is what can be deemed discriminative and organisational abuse, self-neglect, domestic abuse, human trafficking or modern-day slavery, where abuse occurs during the provision of NHS-funded care, including abuse that results in a Serious Case Review or Safeguarding Adult review/enquiry, where delivery of NHS-funded care caused or contributed towards the incident. 'Never events' are defined as 'serious incidents that are wholly preventable because guidance or safety recommendations that provide strong systemic preventative barriers are available at a national level and should have been implemented by healthcare providers' (NHS Improvement, 2018).

In stating that 'awareness of medical harm and efforts to reduce it are as old as medicine itself', the pioneer of patient safety, Professor Charles Vincent, emphasised that 'medical error and patient harm are now acknowledged and discussed publicly by healthcare professionals, politicians and general public' (Vincent, 2010). This more candid outlook has continued till today. This should provide nurses a more insightful understanding of how essential it is for their employing organisation to manage patient safety and serious incidents; thus, the nurse's working knowledge of these is essential. Such matters, which concern an NHS provider's serious incident processes, may involve the police if a crime is suspected, or could be dealt with by the civil courts if compensation through litigation is being sought. Hence, the nurse may find themselves being part of a formal investigation, and like many others, may need to provide written statements, which could be used as evidence for legal purposes. The nurse may also be called to a hearing, Coroners Court, civil or criminal court and be placed under cross-examination by legal representatives. This is an extended aspect of the nurse being legally accountable as an independent practitioner, even within the broader corporate legal responsibilities of the NHS or an independent healthcare provider organisation.

References

Baker, R, 2005. The Shipman Enquiry fifth report: are there lessons for other countries? Quality in Primary Care 13 (1), 1–2.

Barr, J, Dowding, L, 2016. Leadership in healthcare, 2nd ed. Sage, London.

Buka, P, 2015. Patient's rights, law and ethics for nurses. CRC Press, London.

Care Quality Commission, 2015. Regulation 20: Duty of candour. information for all providers: NHS bodies, adult social care, primary medical and dental care and independent healthcare. Available at: www.cqc.org.uk/sites/default/files/_duty_of_candour_guidance_final.pdf.

Caulfield, H, 2005. Vital notes for nurses: accountability. Blackwell Publishing, Oxford.

Concise Oxford English Dictionary, 2011. 12th ed. Oxford University Press, Oxford.

Department of Health, 2000. An organisation with a memory: learning from adverse events in the NHS. London: The Stationery Office.

Francis R, 2013. Report of the Mid Staffordshire Foundation Trust public inquiry: executive summary. The Stationary Office. Available from: https://www.tsoshop.co.uk.

Herring, J, 2020. Medical law and ethics, 8th ed. Oxford University Press, Oxford.

National Patient Safety Agency, 2004. Seven steps to patient safety: the full reference guide. Available at: www.npsa.nhs.uk.

NHS England, 2015. Serious incident framework: support learning to prevent recurrence. Available at: https://www.england.nhs.uk/patient-safety/serious-incident-framework/.

NHS Improvement, 2018. Never events policy and framework. Available at: www.england. nhs.uk and https://improvement.nhs.uk/documents/2265/Revised_Never_Events_policy_ and_framework_FINAL.pdf.

Nursing and Midwifery Council, 2018a. The code: professional standards of practice and behaviour for nurses, midwives and nursing associates. Available at: https://www.nmc.org. uk/globalassets/sitedocuments/nmc-publications/nmc-code.pdf.

Nursing and Midwifery Council, 2018b. Future nurse: standards of proficiency for registered nurses. Available at: https://www.nmc.org.uk/globalassets/sitedocuments/standards-of-pro-ficiency/nurses/future/-nurse-proficiencies.pdf.

Nursing and Midwifery Council, 2020a. What is fitness to practise? Available at: https://www. nmc.org.uk/concerns-nurses-midwives/dealing-concerns/what-is-fitness-to-practise/.

Nursing and Midwifery Council, 2020b. FTP library: understanding Fitness to Practise. Available at: https://www.nmc.org.uk/ftp-library/.

Sullivan, E J, Garland, G, 2010. Practical leadership and management in nursing. Pearson, London.

Supreme Court, 2017. Press summary. Available at: https://www.supremecourt.uk/cases/ docs/uksc-2016-0213-press-summary.pdf (25/1017).

The Shipman Enquiry Fifth Report (2004). Safeguarding patients, lessons from the past – proposals for the future. Command paper, Cm 6394, Stationery Office.

Vincent, C, 2010. Patient Safety, 2nd ed. Wiley-Blackwell & BMJ Publishing Group, Chichester.

Wheeler, H, 2012. Law, ethics and professional issues for nursing: a reflective and portfolio-building approach. Routledge, London.

STATUTES

Employment Rights Act 1996
Health and Safety at Work Act 1974
Health Professions Order 2001
Health and Social Care Act 2008 (Regulated Activities) Regulations 2014
Nursing and Midwifery Order 2001
National Health Service (Concerns, complaints and redress arrangements) (Wales) Regulations 2011

CASES

Bolam v Friern Hospital Management Committee [1957] 1 WLR 583
Bolitho v City and Hackney Health Authority [1998] AC 232 HL
Council for Healthcare Regulatory Excellence and Nursing and Midwifery Council and another [2011] EWHC 927 (Admin)
Ivey v Ghenting Casinos [2017] UKSC 67
Parkinson v Nursing and Midwifery Council [2010] EWHC 1898 (Admin)
Maynard v West Midlands RHA [1985] 1 All ER 635
R v Ghosh [1982] Q.B. 1053
Sidaway v Board of Governors of the Bethlem Royal Hospital and the Maudsley Hospital [1985] AC 871

An Ethical Framework for Nursing

KEY TERMS

Utilitarianism
Deontology

Beauchamp and Childress's
Principles-based approach

Introduction

Throughout their career, nurses are faced with complex and morally challenging dilemmas. The questions that such dilemmas raise for the nurse require answers about what is morally acceptable or what is ethically correct. These questions can be as challenging as the actual dilemmas of clinical practice. As such, the decisions made are based upon the nurses' own judgements and ability to understand moral conflict and be receptive to the patient and significant others who are impacted by the outcomes (actions) of such medical and nursing decisions. Numerous court cases have been decided through moral analysis; as Avery (2013) notes, '…it is the lawyers who can frame the strongest moral argument that will win the day'. This chapter gives a concise introduction to key approaches to ethical reasoning relating to healthcare, with particular emphasis on what is arguably the most influential approach currently – the 'four principles' framework.

Utilitarianism (Consequentialist) Ethics

Act utilitarianism is a form of consequentialist theory, in which an act, in comparison to other acts, is morally right if it bears the greatest possible balance of good consequences and the smallest balance of bad consequences. Herring (2020) describes this as: '…if faced with two alternative courses of action you should choose the one which has the best overall consequences. You should consider each person who may be affected and be sure not to count one person's interests as more important than another's'. Thus, utilitarianism considers everyone's happiness equally, positing that happiness through pleasure is what has intrinsic value, and that actions are 'right' to the extent that they promote happiness and 'wrong' if they produce unhappiness. Although this approach may seem common-sensical, its application in the real world and to medical/nursing practice can be complex. For example, Herring (2020) raises the following questions: what is good? How can you judge how to act if you do not know whether those affected will regard themselves as benefitting (or being harmed) by your actions? Additionally, a consequentialist approach often encounters the unpredictability of not knowing what the consequences of one's own actions are going to be and whether motivation has any relevance in ethical decision-making, if acts are viewed as either 'right' or 'wrong' (Herring, 2020). The belief that everyone's happiness should be counted equally may well be an ideal goal; however, one could ask, if most of the patients in a hospital ward are content and satisfied with their care and progress in reality, how does the utilitarian belief address those patients who are dissatisfied and not progressing?

Rule utilitarianism diverges from act utilitarianism in that its key principle is to follow rules and codes that result in the greatest good for the largest number of people. Whereas 'act' utilitarianism applies the utilitarian principle to individual acts, 'rule' utilitarianism posits that utility can be best considered and extended only by having rules within a moral code; once these rules are established, individual actions can then be judged on the basis of whether they follow these rules. Seedhouse (1998) asserts that *rule utilitarianism* '…argues that obedience to rules, not personal judgement, is fundamental to morality… that rules of conduct are to be worked out by discovering which, if always adhered to, will produce the greatest balance of good over evil'. The utilitarian approach considers that 'good' in a patient (e.g. freedom from disease or harm) needs to be measured in qualitative and quantitative terms, and that short-term consequences of medical and nursing intervention must also consider the possible long-term effects. A hypothetical example would be that of a clinical decision to prolong a patients' life expectancy, reducing the harmful effects of their serious illness by administering a new and/or different medical treatment. However, if this results in their reduced physical and mental abilities, then their quality of life may subsequently deteriorate. Emphasising the importance of estimating the consequences of clinical decisions, Robinson and Doody (2021) assert that just because something benefits 50.5% of the population does not make it good, as it might disadvantage the other 49.5% – 'what is good for one group may not be good for another'.

The well-noted case of twins Mary and Jodie (Case study 4.1) provides an example of a utilitarian decision that illustrates an ethical dilemma faced by doctors, which resulted in a deliberate loss of a patient's life.

The case of the conjoined twins M and J is discussed further in Chapter 9 in relation to the rights of children and medical decision-making.

CASE STUDY 4.1	**(Re A (minors) (conjoined twins: separation) [2000] Lloyds Rep. Med. 425.)**

Conjoined twins Mary and Jodie (M & J) were joined at the lower end of their spines. Their parents appealed against a decision to allow an operation to surgically separate them, which resulted in the death of M. M had severe brain abnormalities and shared a common aorta with J, which rendered her dependent upon J for her blood supply. J had relatively normal functioning and was capable of surviving independently. However, without a surgical separation, the prognosis was that both twins would die within a few months, as supporting M's body would place too much effort on J's. Deeply religious, both parents refused to consent to the separation operation, despite the hospital wanting to carry out the surgery. The parents believed that it should be left to God to decide what should happen to the twins. The doctors applied to the court for a declaration that it would be in the best interests of both twins and lawful to operate. In granting this declaration, the court referred to *Airedale NHS Trust v Bland*, making the analogy to a medical practitioner removing life-sustaining treatment from a patient with no expectation of recovery. Although the parents appealed against the judge's findings, the Court of Appeal dismissed their objections. The principle of best interests moved towards the principle of necessity, of which the following three requirements had been applied to ensure that murder would not be committed: (a) The act (surgery) was required to avoid inevitable and irreparable evil; (b) the steps undertaken were no more than reasonably necessary to accomplish the purpose; and (c) the evil inflicted was not disproportionate to the evil avoided.

Deontological Ethics (*deon* = Greek for 'duty')

Deontology embraces the view that 'certain kinds of actions are good, not because of the consequences they produce, but because they are good and right in themselves' (Herring, 2020) and that '…some duties are… of supreme and abiding importance' (Seedhouse, 1998). Deontology is a rule-based approach to ethics with an emphasis on respecting the moral rules themselves; that is, people have a duty to do the right thing even if it produces a bad result. Examples of such rules would be that it is wrong to steal, to kill an innocent person, to not be truthful, or, alternatively, that it is right to honour agreements. Therefore, a deontologist should do the right thing even if doing so produces more harm or less good than doing the wrong thing. By applying ethical duties to people in all situations, deontological ethics primarily focusses on a person's intentions; that ethics is placed entirely within our control, even though we cannot predict the consequences of our actions. The quandary of uncertainty is not a problem, as deontology is concerned with an action being 'right', because of which a person should perform it; by contrast, if it is a 'wrong' action, they should not do it. This 'right' and 'wrong' ethos is based on a distinct array of moral rules. Therefore, when a person is faced with a moral choice, they should be able to reach a decision with reasonable certainty.

The advantages of deontology could be that it deals with motives and intentions, and emphasises the value of every person, clearly underscoring that some things should never be done, no matter what beneficial consequences they produce. Conversely, the disadvantages could be that it is too inflexible and unconditional, with no cogent basis. Any occurrence which does not fit the commonly held view concerning 'right' or 'wrong' or 'good' or 'bad' is almost regarded as exempt from appraisal or reasoning, and this view may lead to actions that are considered to be less beneficial.

A part of deontology is linked to religion, known as the 'divine command' factor. It emphasises that people should act, live and make moral decisions based on the pronouncements of the divinity, for example, God and the Christian faith's Ten Commandments, and Allah and Islam's Surah Al-An'am. This creates what is known as natural law, which significantly differs from man-made laws, such as case laws and statutes. Thus, it is essential for the nurse to understand and accept that many patients would have strong religious and cultural beliefs they have followed throughout their lives, which will influence their views and decision-making concerning their own care and treatment. The case of *Re T (Adult: Refusal of Medical Treatment)* illustrates a Court of Appeal decision regarding the influence of patient autonomy and informed decision-making on religious grounds.

From a medical and nursing perspective, a deontological approach makes it difficult to reconcile and/or resolve conflicting duties if two professionals morally disagree about the rights and obligations of their clinical reasoning. Herring (2020) argues that consequentialists can debate with each other about the benefits and disadvantages of acting in a particular way. However, there seems no way forward for deontologists who are in disagreement.

Principles-Based Ethics

A popular and influential approach to bio-ethics and healthcare is that of the principles-based approach, developed by American philosophers Thomas L Beauchamp and James F Childress. Their landmark textbook, *Principles of Biomedical Ethics*, was first published in 1979. Their theories and writings have continued to develop, and have received international recognition by doctors, healthcare professionals and academics. Their approach is founded upon four main principles, which need to be considered when dealing with moral issues; it could be regarded as forming a collective moral language with moral commitments. The principles are as follows (Beauchamp and Childress, 1989):

- *Respect for autonomy* – The right of an individual to decide for themselves.
- *Non-maleficence* – Obligation to not harm others.
- *Beneficence* – Obligation to promote the well-being of others.
- *Justice* – Obligation to treat others fairly.

Corresponding with the four principles, Beauchamp and Childress address virtues ethics by highlighting the six essential virtues required for medicine and nursing: care, compassion, discernment, trustworthiness, integrity and conscientiousness. These virtues are not dissimilar to NHS England's six 'C's of nursing (Department of Health, 2012). Again, the importance of values in clinical professions cannot be underestimated. Virtue ethics is a type of normative ethics that emphasises a person's character as the vital element of ethical thinking, rather than rules about actions (deontological) or their consequences (utilitarian). Hence, as Sellman (2017) notes, there is an 'assumption that a person of good character will tend to behave in ways that are consistent with their character'. Beauchamp and Childress (2013) distinguish between personal and professional virtues, in that professional virtues tend to derive from professional standards and employer expectations.

An interpretation of Beauchamp and Childress' essential virtues could begin by noting that nursing is about 'taking care of' and providing 'due care'. Compassion means to have an active and direct regard for the patient's welfare in an empathic and compassionate manner. The nurse should be motivated and try hard to do what is right – being conscientious. However, as Avery (2013) points out, '...the nurse who gives care out of a sense of duty rather than genuine compassion may still be of value to the service, but does not demonstrate the virtue expected of him/her. A discerning approach is to be able to understand the patient's needs and distinguish between the nurse's own anxieties and personal attachments as well as outside influences, thus being able to make the right decisions about the care required'. Moreover, the care of a patient's health can be more effective if the patient is confident regarding the nurse's moral character, competence and integrity. Such integrity includes objectivity, impartiality, reliability, faithfulness to moral values and an awareness of wrongful conduct in clinical practice (Avery, 2013).

The Principle of Respect for Autonomy

Derived from the Greek *autos* (self) and *nomos* (rule, governance or law), autonomy refers to the capacity of an individual to make an informed and uncoerced decision about their future. It respects an individual's choice based on their own values and beliefs. From a nursing perspective, this implies that a patient has a right to decide whether to accept or refuse medical treatment or nursing care, even if the refusal would lead to the deterioration of their health. Beauchamp and Childress (2013) state that personal autonomy incorporates '...at a minimum, self-rule that is free from both controlling interference by others and from certain limitations such as an inadequate understanding that prevents meaningful choice... A person of diminished autonomy, is in some respect controlled by others or incapable of deliberating or acting on the basis of his or her desires and plans'. The three components of autonomy described by Gillon (2003) encompass the self-rule concept succinctly:

- The ability and tendency to think for oneself.
- To make decisions about oneself regarding the way one wishes to lead one's life based on that thinking.
- To enact such decisions.

Operating alongside the self-determination of autonomy is that of the individual being able to govern themselves and live life by their own rules and values (Buka, 2015). However, there are instances where clinicians may well interfere with patient autonomy and question the patient's choices by means of legitimate persuasion intended to be non-coercive; for example, with those suffering from diminished or fluctuating capacity, such as patients with dementia, for whom minimising the risk of harm is imperative. Here, a 'middle ground approach' may respect patient autonomy as well as uphold professional accountability (Greaney and O'Mathuna, 2013). From the perspective of disability, the United Nations Convention on the Rights of Persons with Disabilities (UNCRPD, 2006) asserts the rights of disabled people to have legal capacity on an equal basis with others, and an associated right to make decisions that reflect their own preferences and self-determination. The recognition of such rights by clinicians is conducive to moving away from the traditional notion of 'doctor (or nurse) knows best' towards a more collaborative and less paternalistic relationship that promotes patient autonomy.

The alternative notion of *relational autonomy* is also worthy of consideration. In it, the idea that we live our lives as unconnected individuals is rejected in favour of the view that we base our lives on interdependent relationships (Herring, 2020). In the context of a patient, this may include relatives and healthcare professionals who may work as cooperative partners and be an active part of the patient's decision-making process. Greaney and O'Mathuna (2013) note that relational autonomy 'acknowledges that we do not live in isolation… our decisions reflect our interactions with, and obligations towards, others'. Such obligations would encompass concerns, loyalty, care, friendship and love. Thus, it is necessary for the nurse to be conscious of these dynamics when witnessing or assisting a patient in making decisions about their own medical treatment and welfare.

The Principle of Nonmaleficence

Primum non nocere (Latin: 'first, do no harm') is the obligation to avoid causing harm when actively preventing harm. 'Harm' is a broad term; Beauchamp and Childress (2013) point out the distinction between the notions of 'harming' and 'wronging', in that a person can be harmed without being wronged. For example, contracting a disease or suffering a natural disaster, which are acts for which consent has not been given and occur due to plain bad luck (Beauchamp and Childress, 2013). Conversely, a person can be wronged (e.g. not receive a government welfare benefits payment) without suffering actual harm. Acts of harming are viewed *prima facie* (Latin: 'at first appearance') as wrong, in that they set back, thwart or defeat the interests of the person affected; however, harmful actions that involve 'justifiable' setbacks to another's interests are not wrong (Beauchamp and Childress, 2013). An example of the latter would be that of a patient pursuing a claim for injuries upon a hospital's failure in duty of care, and consequently, receiving a financial sum on grounds of proven negligence. This would be deemed a 'justifiable setback' for the hospital, cause by the legally right action of the patient as a claimant. In explaining that 'harms' include physical pain, disability, suffering, death and mental harm, Beauchamp and Childress (2013) state that the principle of nonmaleficence supports specific *prima facie* moral rules, such as 'do not kill', 'do not cause pain or suffering', 'do not incapacitate', 'do not cause offense' and 'do not deprive others of the goods of life'. Clearly, the related subject of clinical negligence has a distinct link to the principle of nonmaleficence, in that a hospital and its individual clinical workers, such as nurses, owe a duty of care to their patients. A nurse may harm a patient or place them at risk

without malicious or harmful intent, Nevertheless, such wrongdoing and any resulting harm could well result in recourse by the patient and/or their relatives or next
of kin to civil law action, such as financial compensation. Matters such as religious
traditions, professional codes, guidelines, philosophical discourse and the law have
considerable influence upon rules governing non-treatment (e.g. withholding and
withdrawing life-sustaining treatment) and in promoting non-maleficent practice.
The subject of clinical negligence is detailed in Chapter 5, but a technical distinction
between reckless and inadvertent is made by Beauchamp and Childress (2013), in
that negligence can either be '*reckless*', meaning intentionally imposing unreasonable
risks of harm, or '*inadvertent*', that is, unintentionally but carelessly imposing harm.
Many patients enter hospital and leave with additional problems, such as deformity
resulting from surgery, loss of healthy function in parts of the body, wound infections and hospital-acquired infections (e.g. MRSA). Harm-prevention through
education and improving medical intervention and nursing practice is, thus, essential for upholding the principle of nonmaleficence. As mentioned, harm is a broad
term, and a balanced judgement must be made, considering the fact that in the best
interests of a patient, some harm may occur for the greater, long-term benefit.

Numerous healthcare treatments may cause some harm, but may reflect the benefits regarding the outcome of needing to provide such intervention. For example,
blood tests for diagnosis and monitoring of serious illness, or immunisation to prevent COVID-19 infection. Both of these require the use of a hypodermic needle,
which may cause some degree of pain for the patient.

The Principle of Beneficence

The use of the term 'beneficence' in the four principles approach broadly implies 'all
forms of action intended to benefit other persons' and declares a 'moral obligation to
act for the benefit of others'; it differs from *benevolence*, which refers to the personal
quality of 'being disposed to act for the benefit of others' (Beauchamp and Childress,
2013). Beneficence is another *prima facie* principle stemming from the utilitarian
school of philosophy; Beauchamp and Childress make a distinction between *obligatory* beneficence and *ideal* beneficence; that is, we are not morally obliged to benefit
persons on all occasions, but the principle of *ideal* beneficence validates a range of
moral rules of obligation; for example, 'protect and defend the rights of others', 'help
persons with disabilities', 'rescue persons in danger' and 'remove conditions that will
cause harm to others' (Beauchamp and Childress, 2013). The distinctions between
rules of beneficence and nonmaleficence are presented in Table 4.1.

As mentioned earlier, when discussing autonomy, beneficence may be viewed as
veering towards medical paternalism. However, Brazier and Cave (2016) challenge
this notion on the grounds that beneficence demands respect for autonomy; a professional clinician would offer their judgement on what is 'good' for the patient, but
'doing good' for the patient requires that they ultimately accept the patient's decision.

Wheeler (2012) highlights the NHS Trusts' principle of having to balance patient
benefits against risks and financial costs, noting that there will be instances where it

TABLE 4.1 ■ The distinction between rules of beneficence and nonmaleficence

Beneficence	Nonmaleficence
Are positive requirements of action (what should be done)	Are negative prohibitions of action (what not to do)
Prompt the nurse to help the patient and contribute to their welfare	Prompt the nurse not to intentionally inflict harm upon the patient
Need not be followed impartially	Must be followed impartially
Generally, does not provide reasons for punishment by law if agents fail to abide by them	Provision of moral reasons for punishment by law for certain forms of conduct
Adapted from Beauchamp and Childress (2013)	

will not be possible to provide certain treatments, including those in which an NHS Trust is unable to afford the best and most effective treatment. Under the principle of beneficence, even though the trust may choose a less expensive and arguably, not the best treatment, it must be seen to benefit the patient upon considering the scarcity of resources. Additionally, treatment that is unlikely to benefit the patient should not be chosen. Wheeler (2012) refers to the case of *R v Cambridge Health Authority* to illustrate an ethical dilemma that healthcare providers encounter and make decisions upon; see Case study 4.2.

The case of 'B' illustrates the consequentialist ethical perspective based on serving the majority, which also places demands on the Health Authority's limited budget, even though it is at the detriment of the minority (namely 'B'). It is also an example of how the balance between beneficence and nonmaleficence can manifest as finely drawn and complex in reality and that '...difficult and agonising judgements have to be made as to how a limited budget is allocated to the maximum advantage of the maximum of patients... [which are] not a judgement which the court can make' (*R v Cambridge Health Authority*).

CASE STUDY 4.2	**R v Cambridge Health Authority, ex Parte B (A Minor) (1995) 2 All ER 129, CA.**

'B' was a 10-year-old girl suffering from leukaemia, who, in 1994, received a bone marrow transplant which proved to be unsuccessful. The doctors believed she had only six to eight weeks to live and that further treatment would be inappropriate. B's father gained advice that there was a possible course of treatment which included a further (experimental) transplant and chemotherapy, which stood a 10–20% chance of success and a 4% chance of recovery for B. The total financial cost was estimated to be £75,000. The Health Authority refused to fund the treatment on the grounds that the 'experimental' treatment was not in the patient's best interests and that the financial cost could not be justified due to the minimal prospects of the treatment being successful. The Court of Appeal ruled in favour of the Health Authority and demonstrated its reluctance to become involved in matters of resource allocation.

Other examples of cases where the issue of NHS resources played a key factor include *R v Central Birmingham Health Authority* (cancellation of major surgery in a neonate) and *R v Sheffield Health Authority* (refusal to give infertility treatment).

The Principle of Justice

Beauchamp and Childress (2013) refer to *justice* as pertaining to 'fair, equitable and appropriate treatment in light of what is due or owed to persons'. Injustice concerns 'a wrongful [act] or omission that denies people resources or protections to which they have a right'. In healthcare, such fairness could be deemed to comprise equal distribution of access to medical treatment and related services, such as nursing care, assessment/diagnosis and rehabilitation, all of which depend upon the individual needs of those who use such services, and the level of intervention they require. Beauchamp and Childress make the distinction that this *distributive* justice generally refers to the distribution of all societal rights and responsibilities, including civil and political rights. This is distinct from *criminal* justice, which refers to the just means of imposing a punishment for a crime, as well as from *civil* justice, which compensates for matters of tort, such as a breach of contract.

Ebbeson et al. (2012) succinctly describe the *four principles* perspective as a framework for a 'fair health care system' that incorporates both utilitarian and egalitarian standards. This combines an egalitarian strategy, which emphasises the equal worth of persons and fair opportunity, with a utilitarian approach that emphasises 'maximal benefit' to persons and society. For nurses to practice justice and equity, accepting and valuing individual differences is essential. Thus, nurses need to be aware of each patient's factors and attributes, such as culture, religion, social class, ethnicity, sexuality and linguistic and educational ability. Such awareness should be in tandem with the nurse's working awareness of every patient's right to be treated respectfully and with dignity, and insistence that the patient receive the highest standard of compassionate care which respects their privacy and autonomy. A tangible link between the *justice* principle and nursing values can be observed.

At the level of practice, many thoughts and actions concerning the *justice* ethic may be carried out subconsciously, and personal factors, such as the communication style of the nurse or the likeability factor of the patient, may influence how fairly and equitably the nurse treats the patient. As mentioned earlier, limited resources – financial and/or material – play an important part in decision-making concerning patient treatment and care. However, healthcare workers often have limited powers to control or provide more resources. A less tangible resource is that of the 'time' given by the nurse to the patient; nevertheless, this too is often influenced by the availability of clinical staff, who must cover a vast expanse of treatment and care duties. How then does the nurse provide the time to actively listen and engage in a meaningful social discourse with a patient who is able to communicate? The answer to this question is, naturally, dependent on a number of factors, including workload demands, requirement of their time being shared with more sick or demanding patients, as well as having to undertake other duties, such as documentation and non-clinical administrative activity.

As with other ethical viewpoints and models, Beauchamp and Childress' principles-based approach has not been without criticisms. However, its supporters present a strong argument for its important, continuing contribution to medicine and healthcare. Professor Ranon Gillon (2003a) promotes the four principles approach as a 'widely and interculturally acceptable method for medical ethical analysis'. The four principles approach is 'basically simple' enough for it to be used by everyone and not just academics, and it is 'compatible with the insight offered by other approaches to medical ethics' (Gillon, 2003b). Gillon later confirms the approach as 'universalizable as a *prima facie* set of moral commitments… a basic moral language and a basic moral analytical framework' (Gillon, 2014). This stance was recently endorsed by Veatch (2020), who deemed it a 'definitive tool for bioethical analysis' that provides a 'dominant methodology'. Whatever the argument, there is no doubt that the four principles-based approach is currently the most popular ethics model used to educate pre- and post-graduate nurses.

References

Avery, G, 2013. Law and ethics in nursing and healthcare: an introduction. Sage Publications Ltd, London.

Brazier, M, Cave, E, 2016. Medicine, patients and the law, 6th ed. Manchester University Press, Manchester.

Beauchamp, T, Childress, J, 1989. Principles of biomedical ethics, 3rd ed. Oxford University Press, New York.

Beauchamp, T, Childress, J, 2013. Principles of biomedical ethics, 7th ed. Oxford University Press, New York.

Buka, P, 2015. Patient's rights, law and ethics for nurses, 2nd ed. CRC Press, London.

Department of Health (DH) NHS Commissioning Board, 2012. Compassion in practice: nursing, midwifery and care staff – our vision and strategy. Available at: https://www.England.nhs.uk/wp/content/uploads/2012/12/compassion-in-practice.pdf.

Ebbeson, M, Anderson, S, Pederson, BD, 2012. Further development of Beauchamp and Childress' theory based on empirical ethics. Journal of Clinical Research & Bioethics S, 6 e001.

Gillon, R, 2003a. Four scenarios. Journal of Medical Ethics 29, 267–268.

Gillon, R, 2003b. Ethics needs principles – four can encompass the rest and respect for autonomy should be 'first among equals. Journal of Medical Ethics 29, 307–312.

Gillon, R, 2014. Defending the four principles approach as a good basis for good medical practice and therefore for good medical ethics. Journal of Medical Ethics 41 (1), 111–116.

Greaney, AM, O'Mathuna, DP, 2013. Patient autonomy in nursing and healthcare contexts. In: Scott, P A (Ed.), Key concepts and issues in nursing ethics. Springer International Publishing.

Herring, J, 2020. Medical law & ethics, 8th ed. Oxford University Press, Oxford.

Robinson, S, Doody, O, 2021. Nursing & healthcare ethics, 6th ed. Elsevier.

Seedhouse, D, 1998. Ethics: the heart of healthcare, 2nd ed. Wiley, Chichester.

Sellman, D, 2017. Virtue ethics and nursing practice. In: Scott, P A (Ed.), Key concepts and issues in nursing ethics. Springer International Publishing, Switzerland.

United Nations, 2006. United Nations Convention on the Rights of Persons with Disabilities. Department of Economic and Social Affairs: Disability. Available at: https://www.un.org/development/dosa/disabilities/convention-on-the-rights-of-persons-with-disabilities.html/.

Veatch, RM, 2020. Reconciling lists of principles in bioethics. Journal of Medicine and Philosophy 45, 540–559.

Wheeler, H, 2012. Law, ethics and professional issues for nursing: a reflective and portfolio-building approach. Routledge, London.

CASES

R v Cambridge Health Authority, ex Parte B (A Minor) (1995) 2 All ER 129, CA.
R v Central Birmingham Health Authority ex parte Walker [1987] 3 BMLR 32.
Re A (minors) (conjoined twins: separation) [2000] Lloyds Rep. Med.425.
Re T (Adult Refusal of Medical Treatment) [1992] 4 All ER 649, CA
R V Sheffield Health Authority ex parte Seale [1994] 25 BMLR 1

The Tort of Negligence

KEY TERMS

Duty of care
Vicarious liability
Causation
Negligence
Injury

Damage and compensation
Foreseeability
Manslaughter
Expert witness

Introduction

Whilst all clinical practitioners owe their patients a duty of care, a healthcare provider organisation is vicariously liable, with overarching responsibility for and control over the actions of the clinicians it employs. It could be argued that medical negligence claims ultimately promote accountability among healthcare providers, motivating them to improve both patient safety and better working conditions for their clinicians. In the year 2020/21, 12,629 clinical negligence claims were reported in the National Health Service (NHS), and a total of £2,209.3 million were paid-out to settle such claims (NHS Resolution, 2021). When patients who use healthcare services are adversely affected, they may simply want a transparent explanation of what went wrong, and, in some cases, an apology; a health provider's complaints system can address those concerns. To this end, healthcare providers are required to have complaint arrangements. Additionally, following the Care Standards Act 2000 and the Health and Social Care

Act 2008, the power of inspecting and monitoring both NHS and independent care providers have been given to the Care Quality Commission, which monitors the systems that deal with patient complaints. More recently, government-driven protocol has recommended that patients and their legal advisers try and work closely with healthcare providers to resolve disputes without recourse to litigation.

The Duty of Care

In redressing a failure to provide adequate duty of care and matters concerning compensation for the victim of such a failure, Goudkamp and Nolan (2020) describe two principles of the law of tort that are generally applied to accidental injury to person or property: (1) 'that the victim of accidental injury or damage is entitled to redress through the law of tort, if, and only if, his loss was caused by the fault of the defendant or for those whose fault the defendant must answer, and (2) that the redress due from the defendant whose liability is established should be "full" or should, in other words, be as nearly as equivalent as money can be to the claimant's loss'. Lunney et al. (2017) assert that in assuming that the tort of negligence is preceded on fault, 'it must be shown that the defendant was in breach of his duty to take reasonable care of the claimant – assuming such a duty to exist'. The traditional definition of *negligence* dates back to 1856 in *Blyth v Birmingham Waterworks Co*, where the judge explained *negligence* as an '…omission to do something which a reasonable man, guided upon those considerations which ordinarily regulate the conduct of human affairs, would do, or doing something which a prudent and reasonable man would not do'. The recognition of a standard of care has been described earlier (Chapter 3), and the duty of such care was clearly established in *Sidaway v Bethlem Royal Hospital*; that is, a nurse discharging their duty of care implies that they are able to demonstrate that they have exercised 'skill and judgement in the improvement of the physical and mental condition of the patient'. However, the failure of the duty principle was formed through the landmark *Donoghue v Stevenson* common law appeal case in 1932 (see Case study 5.1 below), which evolved from a moral sense of obligation, in which the 'neighbour principle' was established and

---

CASE STUDY 5.1   **Donoghue v Stephenson [1932] AC 562**

Mrs Donoghue went to a café with a friend. The friend brought her a bottle of ginger beer and an ice cream. The ginger beer came in an opaque bottle such that the contents could not be seen. Mrs Donoghue poured half the contents of the bottle over her ice cream and also drank some from the bottle. After eating part of the ice cream, she poured the remaining contents of the bottle over the ice cream and a decomposed snail emerged from the bottle. Mrs Donoghue suffered personal injury as a result, and commenced a claim against the ginger beer manufacturer. The manufacturer was held liable as the duty of care was breached by omitting to clean the bottle, thereby allowing a slug to crawl into it. The consumer (Mrs Donoghue) of the contaminated ginger beer was thus able to sue and recover damages as she suffered a 'reasonable and foreseeable' consequence in vomiting and becoming ill.

where the House of Lords stated '…you must take reasonable care to avoid acts or omissions which you can reasonably foresee would be likely to injure your neighbour'. This consumerist principle then became applicable to the healthcare relationship between clinician and patient as 'neighbours' in law.

The four elements a claimant must overcome when pursuing a claim for negligence are:

- The persons being sued owed the claimant a duty of care.
- The persons being sued breached that duty of care.
- The breach of that duty of care caused the claimant harm.
- The harm (loss/damage) was foreseeable.

It must be noted that the onus of proof is upon the claimant and the standard of proof is, in every practical sense, on the balance of probabilities. Even if a claimant successfully overcomes the hurdle of proving a breach of the duty of care, they must prove that such a breach actually caused them harm, and that the harm/injury was caused by the negligence of the doctor or other care professionals. The tort of negligence is common law that has developed over many years from the outcomes of specific cases (known as 'precedents'); it continues to evolve, though many old cases are important and may still be applicable today.

Vicarious Liability

The word 'vicarious' means 'delegated' (Concise Oxford English Dictionary, 2011). Delegated liability implies the liability that the employer, such as an NHS Trust or private nursing home, may incur for the damage caused to the patient by the negligence of one of its employees, and by whether the employee's act/omission was specifically authorised by the employer. Patients in hospitals are treated by the employees of the hospital or Trust; as such, patients have no say in the selection of the doctor or health professional who is to treat and care for them. Thus, the employer is liable, as it selects its employees and assigns the duties and responsibilities to them. Furthermore, if the care is provided by a private hospital provider, the clinician-patient relationship is overseen by a contract of services. Under contract law, the Trust employing the nurse would pay for damages of negligence upon the principle of vicarious liability. However, if an investigation reveals misconduct, the nurse can be held accountable through reasonable disciplinary measures. Such a breach of the nurse's contract of employment could lead to disciplinary action, and in more serious cases, termination. Therefore, a nurse would be well advised to seek further indemnity cover and legal representation (if attending tribunal or court) through a trade union or professional body, such as the Royal College of Nursing. The concept of vicarious liability originates from the Roman times and was established in English common law in the 16th century. Historically, the master was liable for the acts of his slave/servant, who were undertaken at the master's command; the wrong of the servant was commanded by the master, who was held liable as if the master had commanded the particular act complained of. Case study 5.2 (below) of *Bull v Devon AHA* illustrates such liability.

CASE STUDY 5.2	**Bull v Devon Area Health Authority [1993] 4 Med LR 117**

A woman delivered twins at an NHS hospital that did not have an appropriately qualified obstetrician to deal with the emergency complications of delayed labour. The second child suffered asphyxiation that resulted in a severe disability. Another hospital of the Health Authority had the required obstetrician; however, they were unable to attend in time. The hospital's defence was that in view of the available limited resources, the delay was unavoidable. The mother sued the hospital because of a systems failure.

Bull raised issues concerning adequate skilled medical cover, lack of medical and nursing accountability and the poor quality of unreliable nursing records, which should have been able to help determine the truth of what occurred. On the premise that hospitals and health authorities have a duty of care, and that they may be liable for an inadequate system which places the responsibility of care under staff members who may be designated appropriate but not competent, Brazier and Cave (2016) posit that such 'systems errors' would imply that action should be made directly against the hospital. A later case of *Child A v Ministry of Defence* reinforced the liability of an organisation that fails to ensure that hospital staff and facilities are 'appropriate to provide a safe and satisfactory service'. In this case, A's father was a military serviceman posted to Germany accompanied by his wife – A's mother. A was born in a German hospital, but suffered brain injury at birth. His mother sued the Ministry of Defence (MOD). The designated German hospital had been contracted via an English hospital by the MOD to provide healthcare for servicemen and their families; consequently, the MOD was deemed to have a duty of care.

Breach of Duty of Care

If *Bolam* remains the objective test for a defendant failing to reach the expected standard of care, then, as mentioned in Chapter 3, it is essential to understand the case of *Bolitho v City and Hackney Health Authority* (Case study 5.3). This case extended *Bolam* in terms of medical practice being accepted as proper from a 'responsible body of medical opinion' that informs standards of care. *Bolitho* heralded a move from 'responsible' to 'respectable', highlighting that the courts expect logical decision-making to be observed, in which risks are weighed against benefits by those giving 'expert evidence', and that a 'defensible conclusion' is reached. A 'respectable' practitioner is someone with an extra standing within a profession; such practitioners may be called to provide independent evidence as experts within their own field. Following *Bolitho*, evidence-based practice and the use of expert witnesses has played a greater role in determining negligence claims. When there are competing views on the rightfulness of a defendant's conduct, the courts are directed to not simply accept medical opinion, but carefully scrutinise the evidence. However, it is more an exception that a judge rejects medical testimony, which only occurs when such testimony is unreasonable or irresponsible. Nevertheless, as Brazier and Cave (2016) state, the courts, not the medical professionals, are the 'ultimate arbiters' of the standard of care in claims concerning clinical negligence.

CASE STUDY 5.3	**Bolitho v City & Hackney Health Authority [1997] 3 WLR 1151**

A 2-year-old child (Patrick Bolitho) was admitted to a hospital with breathing difficulties. After initially recovering from two episodes, he relapsed. A paediatric senior registrar (defendant) was summoned, but they did not respond. The child suffered cardiac and respiratory arrest, which led to severe brain damage and death. The child's mother brought an action, claiming that the defendant should have attended and intubated, to save her son's life. The defendant stated that even if she had attended, she would not have intubated the child. This view was endorsed by another doctor. Although the defendant was deemed to have breached her duty of care by not attending, the child's death was not deemed to be due to that breach, as the refusal was not illogical. The court stated that it was not possible for a defendant to argue that a breach did not cause the harm, because but for the breach, some other breach would have been committed. In assessing whether the defendant would have been in breach had they attended and not intubated the child, the judge applied the *Bolam* test, where expert evidence was given by other doctors, the majority of whom, upon assessing the clinical presentation of the child, said they would have acted in a similar manner. Thus, the House of Lords accepted that the defendant's practice was logical, defensible and in accordance with practice accepted as proper by a responsible body of medical professionals. The defendant was acquitted at both the trial and Court of Appeal and was not found liable.

Cases of significance in which the courts took a more pre-emptive approach to interpreting medical testimony include: *Marriot v West Midlands Health Authority*, regarding a risk analysis approach, contrary to expert evidence concerning General Practice; *Reynolds v North Tyneside Health Authority*, a midwifery case regarding a body of opinion not being logical or defensible; *Lillywhite and another v University College London Hospitals NHS Trust*, regarding the negligent interpretation of ultrasound in a pregnant woman and failing to identify abnormalities; and *Smith v Southampton University Hospitals NHS Trust*, regarding a Court of Appeal decision where there was a debate upon complex issues in relation to post-surgical complications, and why the court preferred one medical opinion over another.

The Status of Clinical Guidelines

Like other healthcare professionals, nurses are encouraged by national bodies to adhere to guidelines for their clinical practice; an increasing number of public bodies are producing national guidelines. The National Institute for Health and Care Excellence (NICE), which was formed in 1999, may well be the largest body providing authoritative guidance and advice on clinical practice improvement. Such guidance includes the use of best evidence to inform care and meet the standards set by regulatory bodies, such as the Nursing and Midwifery Council (NMC) and the National Health Service Litigation Authority (NHSLA) risk management requirements. Within a legal context, earlier commentary by Hurwitz (1995) addressed whether the guidelines were advisory or mandatory, and what regulatory function they served. Did clinicians have a large enough role for clinical discretion?

In considering such questions, a nurse who may deviate from clinical guidelines during their practice should be taken into account, with regards to how this may place them at risk of being held liable for negligence. Samanta et al. (2006) support the use of well-constructed and authoritative clinical guidelines to establish the standard of care, positing that their use could 'elevate the quality of healthcare and provide doctors with greater certainty of what is expected of them by law'; the same belief could apply to nurses. As independent practitioners, nurses need to consider whether such guidelines are backed by statute, and which guidelines embody clinical practice accepted as proper by a responsible body of nurses or doctors. They should be mindful of not regarding guidelines as quasi-legislations, and be aware that they may have to defend the accepted practice when it is contrary to national standards. Here, the nurses must demonstrate professional judgement and act responsibly with an up-to-date knowledge of their specialist area of clinical practice; consequently, they should be able to justify their actions within whatever protocols they are working with – accountability for thinking and acting.

Causation

Establishing causation is the third stage in a negligence claim, and consists of two parts – *factual* causation, which addresses whether the defendant's negligence had a historical involvement in the harm caused, and *legal* causation, which addresses whether it is appropriate to consider the factual cause (i.e. defendant's negligence) as responsible for the harm, and the scope of the defendant's liability. This scope of liability involves an assessment of the strength and nature of the causal connection between breach and harm, and consideration of the effect of intervening acts, whether from the claimant or a third party, that arose between the defendant's negligence and the claimant's injury. Furthermore, if the harm is too remote, should the defendant have to pay the full scope of compensation?

Proof of causation for injury/damages can be the most difficult for a claimant to successfully pursue a medical negligence claim. The claimant must prove that the defendant's lack of care caused their injuries, based on the balance of probabilities; additionally, even if sufficient causal connection can be proven, the claim may fail if the defendant's breach was too remote and not a cause of the damage in law. The generally accepted approach to establishing factual causation is what has come to be known as the 'but for' test, which originated from the 1952 case of *Cork v Kirby Maclean Ltd*. In this case, concerning an industrial accident of a man who suffered epilepsy, the judge's summary described what is now the foundation of the 'but for' test: '…if the damage would not have happened but for a particular fault, then that fault is the cause of the damage; if it would have happened just the same, fault or no fault, the fault is not the cause of the damage'. The function of the 'but for' test is primarily to eliminate those factors which could not have had any causal effect, and not to assign legal responsibility. The case of *Barnett v Chelsea & Kensington Hospital Management Committee* is commonly referred to as an illustration of the principle behind the 'but for' test, presented in Case study 5.4.

CASE STUDY 5.4	**Barnett v Chelsea & Kensington Hospital Management Committee [1969] 1 QB 428**

Three workmen had drunk tea and become seriously ill. One of them (Mr Barnett) went to the local hospital Accident and Emergency Department with stomach pains and vomiting, and was attended to by a nurse who telephoned the duty doctor. The doctor advised that Mr Barnett be sent home and contact his General Practitioner (GP) the following day. However, he died 5 hours later from arsenic poisoning. Although the doctor had breached his duty of care in not performing an accurate assessment, his breach was not proved to be the cause of Mr Barnett's death, based on the 'but for' test. But for the doctor not attending, would Mr Barnett have suffered the damage he did? It was held that even if the doctor had attended Mr Barnett, he would have died nevertheless. Consequently, the Hospital was not held liable, as there was no causation.

Another example for grasping the essence of the 'but for' test is the more recent case of *Oakes v Neininger and others* concerning the failure of a GP to diagnose the early stages of cauda equina syndrome. The claimant was left with permanent disabilities, including mobility and incontinence problems. The court held that although the GP could not be held responsible for the development of the medical condition, his delay in making a diagnosis and slow ambulance transfer of the claimant to a hospital caused the irreversible injuries. 'But for' the delay, the claimant would have made a full recovery.

For the nurse, issues of proving causation may arise when considering a clinical team's collective responsibility for upholding the standard of care. However, can inexperience mitigate causation in cases where negligence is in question? This was a matter of consideration in *Wilsher v Essex AHA*, where a premature baby was placed in a special care unit and given too much oxygen by a junior doctor, who incorrectly inserted a catheter and caused oversaturation of oxygen. This caused near incurable blindness from retrolental fibroplasia. The junior doctor had asked a senior registrar to check if what he had done was acceptable; however, the senior registrar failed to identify the error. The trial judge found that a junior doctor owes the same standard of care as a senior doctor, but the registrar was found negligent, as the inexperienced junior doctor had discharged his duty to the senior registrar. Nevertheless, the administration of oxygen was only one of the many equal possible causes of the brain damage. Therefore, liability could not be found on the balance of probabilities. The Health Authority appealed, and with the burden of proof laying with the claimant, the Appeal was allowed. Eventually, an out of court settlement was made. The nurse must be mindful not to practice beyond their competence, and be in recognition of their own clinical practice limitations and seek assistance when required. Not only does this have the benefit of getting help from a senior colleague (although in *Wilsher*, the senior colleague made the same mistake), but is also an appropriate discharge of duty of care to the patient. In *Wilsher*, the belief of collective (team) liability was not accepted; therefore, the courts focussed on the individual's responsibility for their error. Another argument for the defence in the case was that the junior doctor was inexperienced and did not have sufficient time to develop skills; as such, some allowances should have been made for this. Again, the court did not accept this on the basis that every patient has the right to a reasonable standard of care, regardless of who is providing that care. Additionally, the act carried out by the clinician is based on the task being performed and not the degree of the clinician's experience. As Herring (2020) comments, 'It should not automatically be thought that it is a defence for a health care professional to say that they were "only following orders" from a senior clinician'.

Material Contribution to Injury

The case of *Garcia v East Lancashire Hospitals NHS Trust*, concerning a new-born child suffering brain damage from a CVA, illustrates the complexities of causation where more than one possible cause of injury exists, in which there was a failure to establish causation. In case of there being more than one possible cause of the damage, only one of which is the defendant's negligence, then it is sufficient if the claimant can prove that the defendant's conduct materially contributed to the claimant's injury, even if the defendant's breach of duty was not the only or major cause of the injury. Lunney et al. (2017) describe this as a 'cumulative causation' in which the breach must have made the injury worse than it would have been otherwise. Following the principle laid down in the landmark case of *McGhee v N.C.B.*, in the case of *Fairchild v Glenhaven Funeral Services Ltd*, claims were filed by workers who had been exposed to asbestos fibres or dust during their working lives, but had worked for different employers, thus being subject to varying degrees of asbestos exposure throughout. See Case study 5.5 (below).

The decision in *Fairchild* was in favour of the claimant through the Appeal Court; in this case, the facts were such that the 'but for' test could not be reasonably applied.

CASE STUDY 5.5	**Fairchild v Glenhaven Funeral Services Ltd [2002] UKHL 22**

Mr Fairchild was one of three claimants who contracted malignant mesothelioma (lung cancer) as a result of their exposure to asbestos during various paths of work with different employers. Notably, once humans are exposed to it, asbestos fibres are latent for 30–40 years in human lungs before causing a cancerous tumour, which could take almost a decade to cause the victim any distressing symptoms. By the time the symptoms appear, the cancer is in a late stage and cannot be treated. A single incident of exposure to asbestos fibres is sufficient to trigger the cancer, and repeated or prolonged exposure has no bearing upon the severity of the disease. Whilst the claimants had all experienced exposure with each employer, they were neither able to demonstrate nor detect through scientific investigations which employer was the most likely source of the causative asbestos fibre. Therefore, it was unclear from which employer, if any, the claimants were entitled to claim compensation from their tortuous negligence in exposing their employees to asbestos. The House of Lords held that where a claimant could satisfy the burden of proof that one employer had materially contributed to their asbestos exposure, thus raising the probability of the claimant contracting cancer, the claimant could claim total compensation from them; that employer may claim shared contributions from other employers. The court believed that in this situation, it would have been fundamentally unjust to reject any remedy for the claimants.

Thus, the 'materially increased risk' of harm test was used. In this instance, the principle adopted was that of *McGhee,* with a formulated stepped approach to determine liability. Where the injury can be divided, the defendant may be liable to the claimant only for that part of the harm that he has proved to have caused. A finding of 'material contribution' is sufficient for the claimant to recover in full if the court is not satisfied that the tort alone is sufficient for the claimant, or if the evidence does not enable the courts to determine any apportionment (Goudkamp and Nolan, 2020). This was the case in *Bailey v Ministry of Defence,* where the Court of Appeal upheld a finding of negligence. A woman had undergone bile duct surgery, which caused heavy bleeding; she received inadequate fluid replacement post-operatively, after which she underwent further surgical procedures. Subsequently, she developed pancreatitis, which caused her to inhale her vomit and suffer a cardiac arrest; consequently, she suffered permanent brain damage. The failure to provide post-op care with adequate hydration was a 'material contribution', as it increased the chances of a cardiac arrest; however, the pancreatitis itself was not the fault of the defendant.

Remoteness and Foreseeability

The legal test for causation (otherwise known as 'scope of liability') depends upon the foreseeability of harm and the test of remoteness. Thus, if the damages are unforeseeable, then it is too remote as a matter of law. Foreseeability implies that the defendant should have been able to reasonably predict that their actions/inactions would lead to a particular consequence. Therefore, if the consequence of a wrongful act could have been foreseen by a reasonable person, they are not too remote. A defendant would not be liable for damages that are outside the scope of liability (too remote), even if their negligence did cause factual harm – failure of duty linked to loss and the type of loss must be substantially likely to arise from the breach. As Lunney et al. (2017) describe, when using the analytical tool called the 'scope of risk' approach, if the claimant's damage falls within certain risks that are created by a defendant, then the defendant may be held liable, as the risk is foreseeable, resulting from the defendant's negligence. Conversely, '…if the damage suffered bears no relation to the risk created, why should the defendant be liable?' Scott (2019) further explains that probability is a matter of degree and that foreseeability serves to qualify probability. In the context of remoteness, it serves as a limiting principle, ruling out liability with regard to risks which the defendant could not have possibly anticipated. This scope of risk approach emanated from the case of *Overseas Tankship (UK) Ltd v Morts Dock & Engineering Co Ltd,* where the 'Wagon Mound' test was developed to assess foreseeable damage, which must be of the same 'kind' as the damage that actually occurred. One exception to the foreseeability rule is the 'egg-shell' (or 'thin-skull') rule, an established principle in law that links causation with quantifying physical damages. It derives from a case in 1901, based on a claimant having a hidden weakness and therefore, a possible susceptibility to injury that a defendant did not know about. Because of negligent action, the claimant's vulnerability made them suffer the damage more instantly, and the defendant was considered responsible for the damage as though the claimant was of normal strength. This was observed in *Reaney v University Hospital of North Staffordshire NHS Trust*.

Loss of a Chance

This is a complex aspect of causation, where a claimant alleges that because of the defendant's negligence, he lost the chance of successful recovery from an injury. According to Turton (2009), the patient may be able to recover a portion of the compensation to represent the 'chance' of recovery that they have lost. However, the following Case studies 5.6 of *Hotson* and *Gregg v Scott* reject this argument, whilst providing illustration of this aspect of the causal process.

Hotson and *Gregg* have been the subject of intensive scrutiny and debate amongst the legal and academic professions, such as what exactly was the patient's loss in *Hotson*. An earlier commentary by Armirthalingam (2003) questioned whether *Gregg* had been an attempt to 'fudge the nature' of the injury by fusing physical

---

CASE STUDY 5.6

HOTSON v EAST BERKSHIRE H.A. [1987] 2 ALL ER 909

A 13-year-old boy fell out of a tree, and sustained fractures to his hip that remained undiagnosed when he was taken to the hospital. Five days later, he returned to the hospital in pain, and an x-ray revealed his injury. Subsequently, he was given treatment, but he suffered a vascular necrosis which left him with a permanent disability and chronic osteo-arthritis. Expert medical testimony submitted that had the boy's hip condition been identified on the initial visit, he would have had a 25% chance of making a full recovery with relevant medical treatment; consequently, the judge awarded 25% of what would have been the full amount as damages. The Hospital appealed, which was allowed by the House of Lords, and the claim failed. It was shown that the claimant had not satisfied the burden of proof in evidencing that on the balance of probabilities, 'but for' the hospital's negligence (a delay), the boy would have had at least a 51% chance of recovery. Thus, even though the hospital's negligence on the initial visit was the cause of the necrosis, it was probably the fall (75% chance) which was the cause.

GREGG v SCOTT [2005] 2 WLR 268

The claimant (Mr Gregg) sought a medical opinion after noticing an unusual lump under his armpit. His doctor incorrectly (and negligently) diagnosed the lump as benign. It was a further nine months before the lump was diagnosed as a malignant cancer. During this time, the claimant's medical condition significantly worsened and the lump had grown considerably. Expert medical opinion suggested that had the lump been correctly diagnosed at the claimant's original appointment, he would have had an approximately 42% chance of survival; however, by the time the lump was correctly diagnosed, the likelihood of his survival decreased to 25%. Furthermore, the delay had restricted the range of treatment options available to the claimant. In citing *Hotson*, the House of Lords, on a majority ruling, upheld the Court of Appeal decision that on the balance of probabilities, the delay in treatment had not been shown as causing the loss. Even though the defendant had been negligent with their initial assessment, it remained that loss of a chance was not a form of injury which could be claimed for damages for tortious negligence relating to medical problems.

damage with the actual loss – the chance of survival, and as to whether loss of chance should be recognised as 'actionable damage'.

Res Ipsa Loquitur (Latin: The Thing Speaks for Itself)

This doctrine is often applied if '…an accident has occurred of a kind that usually only happens if someone has been negligent, and the state of affairs that produced the accident was under the control of the defendant, it may be presumed in the absence of evidence that the accident was caused by the defendant's negligence' (Oxford Dictionary of Law, 2018). First described in 1865 in *Scott v London*, *res ipsa loquitur* holds that if it is self-evident that the defendant has damaged the claimant and that the injury would never have occurred in the normal course of events, it is up to the defendant to prove that their conduct did not injure the patient. However, though *res ipsa loquitur* implies negligence that the defendant must successfully 'rebut', it does not move away from the claimant needing to establish the burden of proof. As Herring (2020) succinctly describes, when the claimant is unable to directly prove medical negligence, they claim that it is obvious from the circumstances and the fact of the injury that there was negligence.

Notable cases where this doctrine has been used include *Glass v Cambridge H.A.*, where a claimant suffered a heart attack whilst under general anaesthetic; *Lillywhite v University College London Hospital's NHS Trust*, where a consultant allegedly failed to detect an obstetric condition; *Sutcliffe v Aintree Hospitals NHS Trust*, concerning contaminated anaesthesia that led to neurological damage; *Thomas v Curley*, where surgery under general anaesthesia resulted in a common bile duct injury; and a private healthcare case of *Hussain v King Edward VII Hospital*, where a shoulder injury emerged following a genito-urinary surgery.

Causation and a Duty to Inform

Negligence concerning a claim based on failure to provide a patient adequate information about proposed treatment, such as the failure to give adequate warning about possible adverse side effects, was the subject of another landmark case – *Chester v Afshar* (Case study 5.7). Here, the claimant had to establish that had the risks of operation been disclosed, they would not have accepted the treatment. This case has been the subject of much debate and discussion, and for the reader, serves as an example of complex factors which often must be considered and presented before the court, of which there is no ready solution.

In emphasising that there was a breach of duty in failing to warn the claimant, the majority (3:2 decision) took the view that the surgeon had caused the loss, because if they had given proper advice, the operation would not have taken place on that particular day but on a different day, possibly at the hands of a different surgeon. Therefore a 'modification' of the traditional 'but-for' test was adopted and the

CASE STUDY 5.7	**Chester v Afshar [2004] UKHL 41**

The claimant (Ms Chester) undertook an MRI scan which revealed protruding spinal discs. She had suffered back pain for 6 years, which became severe and resulted in an inability to walk and a loss of bladder control. The claimant was advised to undergo surgery which carried a 1–2% risk that if it was performed correctly, it could cause cauda equina syndrome, which would worsen the claimant's condition. The consultant neurosurgeon (Mr Afshar) was under a duty to warn her of this risk, but failed to do so. The risk later materialised and the claimant was left with a permanent disability. The trial judge found that the surgeon had failed to warn the claimant of the risk, even though he had not been negligent in performing the operation. The claimant argued that had she been fully advised of this risk, she would have taken time to consider further medical opinion, and the judge concurred. The judge accepted the argument that if the claimant had the operation on another occasion, it might have been successful, and therefore, considered this as sufficient to establish causation – ruling in the claimant's favour. After the Court of Appeal upheld the decision, the defendant appealed to the House of Lords on the grounds of causation, in that she was likely to have consented to the operation and that it carried the same risk even if it had been performed on a different occasion. However, the House of Lords dismissed the appeal on a 3:2 majority decision and decided the claimant could recover for her injuries.

risk was viewed by the surgeons as an innate aspect of the operation and would have been the same in any other case. As summed up by one of the Law Lords, '…the function of the law is to enable rights to be vindicated and to provide remedies when duties have been breached. Unless this is done the duty is a hollow one, stripped of all practical force and devoid of all content…' Conversely, the minority dissenting judges presented the argument as to whether one would have taken the opportunity to avoid or reduce the risk and that it was an extension of the law from Fairchild in that it ignored the requirements to demonstrate causation of the harm inflicted and had actually 'dispensed' the principle of causation, rather than it being a 'modification'. The surgeon's failure to warn the claimant of the dangers did not increase the material risk, as the claimant would have undergone the surgery anyway. A patient's right to be appropriately warned is important; however, it should not be reinforced by providing potentially large damage payments by a defendant whose violation of that right is not shown to have worsened the physical condition of the patient. According to Miller (2012), the dissenting judges' identification of the failure to warn was coincidental to the injury, and also more consistent with a layperson's understanding of the notions of risk, chance and probability.

The more recent case of *Montgomery v Lanarkshire Health Board* also advanced the court's consideration of failing to warn in a case that focussed on the standard of care in the patient's interests, and that risk disclosure is about facilitating the patient's understanding of specific ('technical/clinical') information; it is not just an outcome between doctor and patient (Turton, 2019). The claimant (Mrs Montgomery), during her pregnancy, did not have the risks of delivery and the option of a caesarean section delivery explained to her. Being of small stature and a diabetic, there was likelihood that the foetus would be large, a 9–10% risk of dystocia and a 0.1% risk of cerebral palsy occurring with her new-born child. Unfortunately, this was the outcome. An eventual Supreme Court decision ruled in her favour and awarded damages for negligence. The most significant aspect of the judgement was the shift in the assessment of duty of care, from the medical profession to one that rests on the needs, anxieties and context of the patient, to the extent that they should be known to the doctor. Montgomery is presented in further detail in Chapter 9, when discussing informed consent and the doctor-patient relationship.

Contributory Negligence

Brazier and Cave (2016) ask, 'Could a doctor or a hospital ever plead contributory negligence and argue that the claimant's injury was in part at least his own fault?' In today's consumer-empowered society where people take responsibility for their own health choices, will the defence of contributory negligence become more common if a patient has not attended their hospital out-patient appointment, followed instructions to take prescribed medicine/treatment or heeded advice to stop smoking or modify dietary intake? A claimant may recover much less or no compensation for damages if they were seen as negligent themselves in causing their own harm. The Law Reform (Contributory Negligence) Act 1945 concisely describes its provision:

> '...Where any person suffers as the result of his own fault and partly of the fault of any other persons, a claim in respect of that damage shall not be defeated by reason of the fault of that person suffering the damage, but the damages recoverable in respect thereof shall be reduced to such extent as the court thinks just and equitable having regard to the claimant's share in the responsibility for the damage...'

This is known as the *apportionment provision*. Notably, the Act does not define contributory negligence and defines 'fault' to mean negligence, breach of statutory duty or act/omission which gives rise to liability in tort. The apportionment provides that damages are recoverable at a reduced level due to the claimant's share in the responsibility of the damage. As Goudkamp and Nolan (2020) describe, the judge identify the parties' respective share of responsibility for the damages claimed in terms of percentages and often simply declare the given apportionment in a common-sense way and not scientifically. The case of *Horsley v Cascade Insulation Services & Others* is a relevant example illustrating contributory negligence. It concerns a man who contributed to his disability due to his own lifestyle despite health warnings.

The influence of a break in causation (Latin: *novus actus interveniens*) is worth mentioning briefly. This is where 'An act or event that breaks the causal connection between a civil wrong or crime committed by the defendant and subsequent happenings and therefore relieves the defendant from responsibility for these happenings' (Oxford Dictionary of Law, 2018). Examples would include an intervening natural event which causes damage that is independent of the defendant's breach of duty or the intervening act of a third party, which could range from an innocent mistake to a wilful wrongdoing. Novus actus interveniens requires that the secondary act (or event) was not reasonably foreseeable and disturbs the initial act, whereby the subjective test of legal causation can no longer be satisfied.

Psychiatric Injury

Relatively speaking, the law has a more restrictive approach in awarding damages for psychiatric injury inflicted by negligence. It lays down several hurdles that the claimant must fulfil to establish liability. First, there must be an actual psychiatric injury; sorrow, emotional grief, feelings of fear, panic or terror are insufficient. As the case of *Alcock v Chief Constable of South Yorkshire* affirms, there must be some 'recognisable acknowledged psychiatric illness'. Such an injury draws a distinction between two types of victims: (i) primary – those who are involved or are immediately within the zone of physical danger; and (ii) secondary – those not within the physical zone of danger but witness horrific events. A primary victim only needs to establish that the physical harm was foreseeable; they neither require that psychiatric injury be foreseeable nor do they owe the secondary victim a duty of care in relation to self-inflicted harm. For a secondary victim to establish liability, they must demonstrate that the following four *Alcock* criteria are present:

1. *A close tie of love and affection,* which may be presumed in parent and child or between spouses, but has to be proved in other relationships. Siblings are not usually considered to have a close tie or affection.
2. *Witness the event with their own unaided senses* and not through another medium, such as television or video footage.
3. *Proximity to the event itself or its immediate aftermath* means that it is necessary for the claimant to have a 'close tie of love and affection' with the injured or endangered person and that this requirement of proximity of relationship seems to 'close the door on claims by mere bystanders' (Lunney et al., 2017). The immediate aftermath is decided upon the facts presented within each individual case.
4. *Psychiatric injury must be a result of a shocking event* as described in *Alcock*: '….shock, in the context of this cause of action, involves the sudden appreciation by sight or sound of a horrifying event, which violently agitates the mind. It has yet to include psychiatric illness caused by the accumulation over a period of time of more gradual assaults on the nervous system'.

However, this area of law has been criticised for the judiciary's imprecise, inconsistent approach with a reliance on a psychiatric diagnostic label, for example, Post-Traumatic Stress Disorder. Ahuja (2015) criticises what he describes as the 'archaic principles' of traditional approaches, claiming that the law goes against medical evidence in calculating the evidence for the threshold *Alcock* requirements and that 'distress must be a diagnosable psychiatric disorder to be actionable'. A distinction needs to be made between psychological harm and psychiatric disorder, where psychological harm could include any emotional distress that has some impact on a person's functioning, irrespective of whether it is diagnosed as psychiatric illness, in addition to a belief that a psychological assessment of impact (causing injury) will provide more pertinent answers in this area of law (Ahuja, 2015). Notable court cases which further explore this aspect of negligence include *Re (A Minor) v Calderdale and Huddersfield NHS Foundation Trust*, regarding a claim concerning post-traumatic shock after a dreadful labour and birth, and *Crystal Taylor v A Novo (UK) Ltd*, regarding a failed claim for an event concerning a deceased relative.

Gross Negligence Manslaughter

For negligence to move from civil to criminal law, death of a patient usually has to occur and the professional misconduct of the healthcare professional must be so severe that it significantly contributed to that death – gross negligence manslaughter. Although rare for a clinician to harm a patient deliberately or for manslaughter to take place, increasing cases concerning medical professionals are being brought to the courts for prosecution, particularly since the Corporate Manslaughter and Corporate Homicide Act 2007 and the Criminal Justice and Courts Act (Section 20) 2015 created a new offence of 'ill-treatment' or 'wilful neglect'. The case of a successful prosecution was that of *R v Adomako*, where proof of gross negligence had to satisfy the test of one of the following questions:

- Did the healthcare professional show indifference to the risk of injury to the patient?
- Did the healthcare professional decide to run a risk for no good reason – recklessly?
- Were the healthcare professional's attempts to avoid a known risk so poor to be seen as grossly negligent?
- Did the healthcare professional make no effort to avert a serious risk through inattention or failure to have regard for such a risk?

R v Misra and Srivistava and *R v Prentice* are cases which further illustrate the considerations of manslaughter. In *Misra*, the Adomako test was applied and a conviction made concerning the post-operative death of a patient from toxic shock. *Prentice* concerned a quashed conviction by the Court of Appeal following a fatal injection into a patient of a drug by the incorrect route.

Brazier and Cave (2016) raise the question of what constitutes gross negligence and that the term is vague and vulnerable to subjective interpretation by juries. More recent commentary by Robson et al. (2020) bring together the principles of both civil and criminal law to create better clarity and address the matter of culpability which at the most severe end of the scale results in the death or serious injury of a patient, and which entails the clinician having carried on regardless or ignoring a red flag irrespective of the consequences and with no excuse; this may well amount to an offence of recklessness. In emphasising that a criminal offence of recklessness requires culpability, Robson et al. (2020) view the culpability aspect as being poorly defined. A clinician who acts in good faith, but makes a bad choice where a patient is unlucky enough to die, may be labelled a "criminal", but such a label does not fulfil the requirement of *mens rea* (Latin: the intention or knowledge of wrongdoing) as this is often unclear or absent.

Assessing Damage and Compensation

The purpose of assessing damages is to place the claimant in a position they would have been had they not suffered the harm. Assessment of damages can either be by agreement or by the courts; if there is a loss of limb or permanent brain injury, then a patient who proves negligence is eligible for a compensatory award. Agreement of damages is when both parties attempt to agree on a figure (quantum) that returns the patient as closely as possible to the situation they were in before the harm occurred. If both parties cannot agree, then the courts decide the level of damages for the claimant. Generally, the greater the disability, the higher the award, and the longer the patient has to live with their injuries, the greater the sum of financial compensation. Pursuing claims, however, often take a reactive, defensive and adversarial approach which does not encourage openness (Martin, 2005). It must be borne in mind that the purpose of compensation is restorative, rather than punitive (Avery, 2016). The actual process of assessment and calculation of awards is complex and legislated through the Damages Act 1996 and Damages (Personal Injury) Order 2001, where claimants can either receive a lump sum or a series of payments (Periodic Payment Order) over time. The final sum awarded has to take into account how the claimant will invest and use the money; thus, calculations have to be made upon rates of interest and the assumption that claimants would invest in index-linked financial savings schemes.

Damages awarded to the claimant are divided into pecuniary (financial) and non-pecuniary loss. Non-pecuniary essentially covers pain and suffering attributable to the injury itself and any medical treatment received as a consequence. Loss of amenity is covered, such that where a claimant has been deprived of pleasures that they had previously experienced, he is entitled to damages; for example, being unable to play a sport or loss of sexual ability. In assessing an actual injury, the courts can refer to an arbitrary tariff to calculate the award, which is often based upon similar previous injury claims. This assists in bringing consistency into the decision-making process. By contrast, pecuniary losses cover loss of earnings from paid employment; loss of the capacity to work and earn due to the disability; reduced expectation of life or 'loss of years'; future medical expenses, including equipment or home adaptations. In cases where gratuitous care is required and there is speculative loss of future earnings, what will be the claimant's future medical fees? What would the claimant have earned had they not been injured? The limitation period (time limit) for a person to make a claim is 3 years from the incident or when the injury occurred.

The process of assessing compensation underwent significant reform following the Report on Access to Justice and an overhaul instituted by Lord Woolf in 1999, mainly that of the code of the Civil Procedure Rules (Ministry of Justice, 2021). One significant change was that parties were encouraged to resolve matters of dispute before going to court, using mediation or alternative dispute resolution. This became more imperative since the removal of legal aid for claimants and the introduction of conditional ('no win – no fee') systems into civil litigation. In summary, the Civil Procedure Rules were intended to maintain justice and proportionality, as well as save expense on court costs, ensuring that cases were dealt with more quickly and efficiently with the introduction of the *pre-action protocol*, which was to set the standard for better handling matters of dispute, including investigation and information management.

The Nurse as Expert Witness

A nurse may be summoned to a criminal, civil or Coroners Court to provide evidence at any time. Furthermore, there are nurses who, through their knowledge and experience, take on an additional function of what is termed an 'expert witness'. Expert witnesses exist across various professions. An expert is generally regarded as a person 'who has received training, possesses qualifications and has obtained significant practical experience in his (her) given field of expertise' (Stockdale, 2014). Expert nursing evidence, as with other forms of evidence, may be required by a court for a number of reasons, such as trying to establish the cause of a patient or victim's death, and the admissibility of evidence in the civil court, which is governed by the statute of the Civil Evidence Act 1972. The expert, following instructions, formulates their own opinion and produces a report (as evidence) before the case is heard in court. They may also attend a pre-court meeting with other experts, in which parties to the civil proceedings are permitted to instruct their own experts, with the court directing a discussion between experts to come to an agreement, which would result in a statement to the court as to whether they agree or disagree but ultimately expert evidence is under the control of the court. Expert evidence is under the control of the court. However, as Stockdale (2014) asserts, though a witness might have given expert evidence in previous proceedings, a court in subsequent proceedings can still rule that the witness is incompetent to give expert evidence and not accept that the expert's opinion is correct. The Civil Procedure Rules 1998 (Part 35) (CPR) details the requirements for experts to adhere to when preparing reports and presenting their expert opinion. These CPR also empower the civil court to direct expert evidence relating to an issue to be taken in the form of a single joint expert (SJE). Although Stockdale (2014) points out that this may be against the wishes of both parties, Solon (2013) emphasises that judges prefer an SJE who can advise all parties so there is only one report and opinion to consider. When the court does not direct that the expert evidence take the SJE approach, it may direct an exchange of expert's reports from all parties concerned, emphasising that these run concurrently. The CPR allow for each party to ask questions about the report to the respective expert, and these answers are treated as part of the report. Irrespective of the existence of the differing interests of the relevant parties, Solon (2013) stresses that the expert's first duty is to the court and that they should be truly independent.

Much academic and legal commentary has advised about the essential qualities for a professional to be a credible and competent expert witness. Burns (2014) describes five essential factors for those who are considering instructing an expert to play a key role in judicial proceedings. See Box 5.1 (below).

The nurse who is considering undertaking expert witness duties, or has been asked to act as an expert in court proceedings, should note that experts are no longer

---

BOX 5.1 ■ Five Essential Factors When Choosing an Expert

1. Must possess qualifications, experience and expertise in a particular field = credibility.
2. Must be able to demonstrate an understanding of court procedures and the Civil Procedure Rules, as well as be skilled in giving evidence under examination and cross-examination.
3. In their evidence, the expert should be independent, objective and impartial in their views, and if necessary, be critical of arguments put forward by their own party.
4. Must be professional in report-writing, CPR rules and courtroom presentation skills.
5. Have undertaken expert witness training from an accredited provider.

_____

Adapted from Burns (2014)

---

immune from negligence claims against them. Hence, those undertaking expert witness duties for the courts or legal professions are well-advised to have their own professional indemnity insurance.

References

Ahuja, J, 2015. Liability for psychological and psychiatric harm: the road to recovery. Medical Law Review 23 (1), 27–52.

Armirthalingam, K, 2003. Loss of chance: lost cause or remote possibility? Cambridge Law Journal 62 (2), 253–255.

Avery, G, 2016. Law and ethics in nursing and healthcare: an introduction, 2nd ed. Sage Publications, London.

Brazier, M, Cave, E, 2016. Medicine, patients and the law, 6th ed. Manchester University Press, Manchester.

Burns M, 2014. The dependable witness. Available at: https://www.newlawjournal.co.uk/.

Goudkamp, J, Nolan, D, 2020. Winfield & Jolowicz: tort, 20th ed. Thomas Reuters, London.

Herring, J, 2020. Medical law and ethics, 8th ed. Oxford University Press, Oxford.

Hurwitz, B, 1995. Clinical guidelines and the law. Journal of Evaluation of Clinical Practice 1 (1), 49–60. Available at: https://pubmed.ncbi.nim.nib.gov/9238557/.

Lunney, M, Nolan, D, Oliphant, K, 2017. Tort law: text and materials, 6th ed. Oxford University Press, Oxford.

Martin, J, 2005. Clinical negligence and patient compensation. Nursing Standard 19 (25), 35–39.

Miller, C, 2012. Negligent failure to warn: why is it so difficult? Journal of Professional Negligence 28 (4), 266–280.

Ministry of Justice (2021). Civil Procedure Rules. Available at: www.justice.gov.uk/courts/procedure-rules/civil.

Oxford Dictionaries, 2018. Oxford dictionary of law, 9th ed. Oxford University Press, Oxford.

Oxford Dictionaries, 2011. Concise Oxford English dictionary, 12th ed. Oxford University Press, Oxford.

Robson, M, Maskill, J, Brookbanks, W, 2020. Doctors are aggrieved – should they be? gross negligence manslaughter and the culpable doctor. Journal of Criminal Law 84 (4), 312–340.

NHS Resolution, 2021. Annual report and accounts 2020/21. HC 387 (15/07/21). Available at: www.gov.uk/official-documents.

Samanta, A, Mello, MM, Foster, G, Tingle, J, Samanta, J, 2006. The role of clinical guidelines in medical negligence litigation: a shift from the Bolam standard? Medical Law Review 14 (3), 183–214.

Scott, H, 2019. The history of foreseeability. Current Legal Problems 72 (1), 287–314.

Solon M (2013). What makes an expert witness? Available at: www.NewLawJournal.co.uk.

Stockdale, M, 2014. Criminal & civil evidence, 15th ed. Northumbria Law Press, Newcastle upon Tyne.

Turton, G, 2009. Factual and legal causation – their relation to negligence in nursing. British Journal of Nursing 18 (13), 825–827.

Turton, G, 2019. Informed consent to medical treatment post-Montgomery: causation and coincidence. Medical Law Review 27 (1), 108–134.

CASES

Alcock v Chief Constable of South Yorkshire [1992] 1 AC 310

Barnett v Chelsea & Kensington Hospital Management Committee [1969] 1 QB 428

Bailey v Ministry of Defence [2008] EWCA Civ 883

Blyth v Birmingham Waterworks Co (1856) 11 Ex Ch 781

Bolitho v City and Hackney Health Authority [1997] 3 WLR 1151

Bull v Devon Area Health Authority [1993] 4 Med LR 117

Chester v Afshar [2005] 1 AC 134

Child A v Ministry of Defence [2004] EWCA Civ 641

Cork v Kirby Maclean Ltd [1952] 2 All E.R. 402

Crystal Taylor v A Novo (UK) Ltd [2013] EWHC Civ 194

Donoghue v Stephenson [1932] AC 562

Fairchild v Glenhaven Funeral Services Ltd [2002] UKHL 22

Garcia v East Lancashire Hospitals NHS Trust [2006] EWHC 2062 (QB)

Glass v Cambridge Health Authority [1995] 6 Med LR 91

Gregg v Scott [2005] 2 WLR 268

Horsley v Cascade Insulation Services & Others [2009] EWHC 2945 (QB)

Hotson v East Berkshire H.A. [1987] 2 All ER 909

Hussain v King Edward VII Hospital [2012] EWHC 3441

Lillywhite and another v University College London Hospitals NHS Trust [2005] EWCA Civ 1466

Marriot v West Midlands Health Authority [1999] Lloyds Rep Med 23

McGhee v N.C.B. [1973] 1 WLR 1

Montgomery v Lanarkshire Health Board [2015] UKSC 11

Oakes v Neininger and Others [2008] EWHC 548 (QB)

Overseas Tankship (UK) Ltd v Morts Dock & Engineering Co Ltd (The Wagon Mound) (No 1) [1961] AC 388

R v Misra and Srivistava [2004] EWCA Crim 2375

R v Prentice [1993] 4 All ER 935

Re (A Minor) v Calderdale and Huddersfield NHS Foundation Trust [2017] EWHC 824

Reaney v University Hospital of North Staffordshire NHS Trust [2014] EWHC 3016

Reynolds v North Tyneside Health Authority [2002] Lloyds Rep Med 453

Scott v London & St Katherine Docks Co [1865] 3 H&C 596

Sidaway v Bethlem Royal Hospital [1985] A.C. 871

Smith v Southampton University Hospitals NHS Trust [2007] EWCA Civ 387

Sutcliffe v Aintree Hospitals NHS Trust [2008] EWCA Civ 179

Thomas v Curley [2013] EWCA Civ 117

Wilsher v Essex Area Health Authority [1988] 1 All ER 871

STATUTES

Care Standards Act 2000
Civil Evidence Act 1972
Damages Act 1996
Damages (Personal Injury) Order 2001
Health and Social Care Act 2008
Law Reform (Contributory Negligence) Act 1945

Confidentiality

KEY TERMS

Confidentiality

Privacy

Access to records

Freedom of Information Act 2000

Caldicott principles

Introduction

The nurse has a duty of confidence under law, their NHS employment contract and the Nursing and Midwifery Council (NMC) Code (Parts 5.1–5.5 2018) to respect a patient's rights to privacy and confidentiality. The view of the General Medical Council (GMC) is that, *'There is no overarching law that governs the disclosure of confidential information. The common law and other laws that require or permit the disclosure of patient information interact in complex ways and it is not possible to decide whether a use or disclosure of patient information would be lawful by considering any aspect of the law in isolation'* (GMC, 2017). In providing some definition between privacy and confidentiality, Beauchamp and Childress (2019) describe confidentiality as a 'branch… of informational privacy' which 'prevents redisclosure of information originally disclosed within a confidential relationship…'. An infringement of a person's right to confidentiality occurs 'only if the person/institution to whom the information was disclosed in confidence fails to protect the information or deliberately discloses it to someone without first party consent' (Beauchamp and Childress, 2019).

Confidentiality – The Doctor, Nurse and Patient

The control of confidential information is a complex aspect of clinical practice that raises a number of ethical challenges. For example, respecting a patient's right to privacy may be complicated by a prevailing duty of care, balanced with acting in accordance with the preference and will of the patient. Disclosure of information to a patient concerning their health condition/diagnosis, treatment and prognosis is a question of professional judgement balanced with the patient's right to know and to exercise their autonomy. Sharing confidential information with another healthcare professional may need to occur to enhance care and achieve an improved outcome for the patient. Similar to doctors, nurses too have considerable power over how they possess and control information about their patients; consequently, they must make difficult judgements about what information the patient needs to know and manage the anguish how a particular information may cause. Thus, this aspect requires careful consideration, as the patient and their carers/relatives may need to receive emotional support when faced with new information, which may initially be taken as bad news. In addressing the healthcare professional's authoritative position of knowledge and the vulnerability of the patient who discloses private information, Robinson and Doody (2021) state that 'people will share or hold back information about themselves during their consultations with health professionals depending or whether or not they trust the healthcare professional, and their belief that the healthcare professional will use the information for the benefit of making a diagnosis and managing the problem'.

Exceptions to Absolute Confidence

Adhering to confidentiality in healthcare is arguably not an absolute requirement; thus, the following exemptions to an absolutist view exist, where consent is given by the patient to such disclosure and where the law requires disclosure and/or in the interests of an overriding public need for disclosure. Confidential patient information can be disclosed 'in the public interest where that information can be used to prevent, detect, or prosecute, a serious crime... [which] will certainly include murder, manslaughter, rape, treason, kidnapping, and child abuse or neglect causing significant harm and will likely include other crimes which carry a five-year minimum prison sentence but may also include other acts that have a high impact on the victim' (Department of Health, 2010). Department of Health (DH) guidance emphasises that public interest does not mean, 'of interest to the public' and that each public interest case should be judged upon its own merit. The key factor in deciding whether to share confidential information is the need to meet the requirements of the European Convention of Human Rights Article 8(2) on the 'right to privacy' regarding necessity and proportionality (DH, 2010).

If, as the NMC Code states, a decision to divulge confidential information is a matter of professional judgement, then it is essential for the nurse to distinguish between the circumstances in which they can decide if it is appropriate to divulge what has been considered 'confidential' and the legal duty to disclose such information. Such exceptions, that justify a breach of confidentiality and disclosure of information are briefly described as follows.

- With <u>explicit consent of the patient</u> or their lawyer, which is only lawful if the mentally capacitated patient knows exactly what information is to be disclosed and who is to receive such information. Under the Data Protection Act (DPA) (1998), the requirements for obtaining such consent from patients implies that they know what and why the information is being disclosed, and are given the opportunity to discuss the matter with a person they trust, ask questions and make a choice within a reasonable period of time. The patient needs to fully understand the documentation they may have to sign, and know that they can refuse or withdraw their consent at any time. The healthcare worker is required to place such consent details within the patient's records.

- For <u>care and treatment purposes,</u> where confidential information needs to be communicated with doctors and other healthcare professionals to serve the best interests of the patient. Patients are usually with information disclosure if it has been made clear why personal health information is documented, shared and accessed by other healthcare professionals. The patient also has the right to access their own records and have their questions answered by the professionals involved in their care.

- <u>Patient's refusal or inability to consent</u>. A patient's refusal to allow disclosure of information to other healthcare professionals involved in the patient's care could result in limited care being provided; in some situations, treatment might not be offered. Patients must be informed that their refusal to allow disclosure of treatment information may have repercussions for their future provision of care and treatment. However, nurses and other healthcare professionals should be aware that such refusals can lead to ineffective or unsafe treatment of patients, thereby hindering effective continuity of care due to the absence of relevant information about a patient's condition and medical history. Where a patient is incapable of understanding information or consenting to disclosure of care, disclosure of care and treatment to the patient's relative or main carer may be considered to be applicable, particularly if the patient lacks capacity and/or is vulnerable and at risk of their health deteriorating further.

- <u>Public interest</u>. Disclosure for the public good when there may be circumstances where the public interest is served by disclosing information, even if no criminal conviction is made. The case of *Woolgar v Chief Constable of Sussex Police* provides a good illustration of this particular issue. The UKCC (now the NMC) sought access to confidential material from the police, which was of '...relevance to the subject matter of an enquiry being conducted by the regulatory body, then a countervailing public interest is shown to exist... and is necessary in the interest of the medical welfare of the country, to keep the public safe, and to protect the rights and freedoms of those vulnerable individuals in need of nursing care'. Protecting a third party and/or detecting and preventing serious crime are other exceptions where disclosure may be required. The nurse needs to exercise careful judgement, particularly where vulnerable persons require protection and a disclosure of confidential information outweighs the public interest in maintaining secrecy of confidential information. This balance can also be applied when a nurse is aware that a patient has committed or intends to commit a crime; in such cases, the seriousness of the crime must be considered in view of the counteracting public interest of

CASE STUDY 6.1	W v Egdell [1990] 2 WLR 471

W (plaintiff), a diagnosed paranoid schizophrenic, was a patient formally detained in a secure psychiatric hospital after pleading guilty to manslaughter on the grounds of diminished responsibility for shooting seven people, five of whom died. Ten years later, his solicitor requested psychiatrist Dr H G Egdell to give a written opinion on W's mental state to prepare for an application to the mental health review tribunal, to transfer W to a less secure facility. However, Dr Egdell's report was not in W's favour, as it highlighted W's continued interest in firearms and home-made explosives. The solicitor withdrew W's application, which impelled a very concerned Dr Egdell to make his report available to the hospital medical director with a view that it be referred to the Home Office, as he felt W was giving a false impression to his own psychiatrists. W sued Egdell on the grounds that he had breached his duty of confidentiality. However, the Court of Appeal, in balancing the public interest of 'confidence' and 'disclosure', ruled in favour of the restricted disclosure of crucial information about W's dangerousness on the grounds of grave concern for public safety.

public safety opposed to maintaining patient confidentiality. Hence, the nurse can be required to disclose information to the courts (by *subpoena*) about their patients on the grounds of necessity and in the interest of justice. The milestone case of *W v Egdell* (Case study 6.1) illustrates the issue of disclosure in the interest of public safety.

The conditions dictating the extent of Dr Egdell's disclosure being liable to be outweighed by public interest was highlighted in an earlier landmark USA Supreme Court case of *Tarasoff v Regents of the University of California*. This case related to a psychologist in whom a client had confided, during psychotherapy, that he intended to kill a woman (Tatiana Tarasoff). Although the psychologist had informed the police, he did not warn Miss Tarasoff or her family, and took no steps to detain the client, thus allowing for his early release from hospital. The client subsequently went on to murder Miss Tarasoff, and the parents of the victim sued the University Hospital on the grounds of negligence. From a nursing perspective, a duty to breach confidentiality also depends upon the legal proximity of the victim to the nurse. For example, if the victim was a close relative of the patient involved with the nurse's care plan or if they were another patient under the nurse's care, then it can be argued that the nurse has a duty to warn the victim. However, if a possible victim is an unknown member of the public whom the nurse does not know, then there is no duty to warn. This issue of legal proximity was a key factor in the case of *Palmer v Tees HA*, in which it was claimed that the Health Authority had been negligent in failing to diagnose the high level of risk of a psychiatric patient discharged from their care. The patient went on to abduct, sexually abuse and murder a child. The parents lost their case against the Health Authority for 'failing to warn', in that the identity of the girl was not known to the authority and that the discharged patient may well have found another victim. Thus, it did not owe a duty of care, even though the psychiatrist could have been viewed as failing to assess the seriousness of the risk by discharging the patient too early. These cases raise the immediate dilemma of identifying the point at which 'dangerousness' typically outweighs protective privilege of patient autonomy and absolute confidentiality.

- Statutory duty to disclose. This is for the purpose of fulfilling legislative requirements, for example: Births and Deaths Registration Act 1953 – notification of births and deaths; Public Health (Infectious Disease) Regulations 1988 – health professionals' notification to local authorities of the identity and address of persons suspected of having a notifiable disease; Abortion Regulations 1991 – doctors notifying the Chief Medical Officer of a termination of pregnancy; Prevention of Terrorism Act 2005 – preventing involvement of individuals in terrorism-related activity; The Coroners and Justice Act 2009 – to establish a more effective and transparent service to victims and the public; Misuse of Drugs Act 1971 – to prevent non-medical use of controlled drugs; Road Traffic Act 1988 Part iii and Motor Vehicles (Driving Licenses) Regulations 1999 – legal framework for standards of physical and mental fitness to drive a motor vehicle.

Confidentiality – An Ethical Perspective

From a consequentialist position, the question of whether it is wrong to breach confidentiality can be determined by the consequences of the breach. One of the consequences could be the loss of the patient's trust in their clinical practitioner, which would perhaps cause them to not access healthcare services in the future. This could be detrimental to the patient's health. Conversely, there may be cases in which where there are adverse consequences of not breaching confidentiality, such as a third party being denied information, which would have serious repercussions for their health and future treatment. Wheeler (2012) emphasises the trust between the healthcare professional and patient, noting that the patient needs '…to feel confident to tell their personal health stories… and grant them access to their bodies for clinical observation, examination and various tests required for accurate diagnoses and treatment'. Any inhibitions may prevent the patient from telling their story, and may result in them withholding potentially critical information concerning diagnosis and treatment. Avery (2013) argues that a breach of confidentiality will damage a patient's confidence in healthcare professionals, making them reluctant to seek medical advice for any future-related problems. Under the deontological position, where ethics of duty and the morality of an action depend on the nature of the action (e.g. harm is unacceptable, irrespective of its consequence), confidentiality would be viewed as the nurse having to respect the principles of individual autonomy (self-governance), privacy, confidentiality and the rights and freedom of the patient to make their own decisions. Thus, it is the rules, motives and quality of the nurse's actions, and not the consequences of such actions, that is the most important. If a patient is unaware of a breach of their confidential health information, then, from a deontological perspective, a wrongdoing has occurred. A virtue ethics approach holds that our character is more fundamental to ethical reflection than individual decisions or actions, just as a virtue-based account of professional-patient relationships will be concerned with the character of both health professional and patient (Messer, 2004). Nurses, like other healthcare professionals, are regarded by patients as being trustworthy. Such a virtue, through the therapeutic relationship between nurse and patient, demands that the nurse should demonstrate that they are worthy of such trust, although there may be certain situations where this can be overridden, for example, in the interest of public safety. Virtue ethics veers the obligation onto the nurse's professional demeanour in respecting the patient's rights to autonomy and privacy. The author would suggest that this virtual approach is akin to a psychological contract where the pledge to respect a patient's privacy and uphold their confidentiality is a fundamental aspect of daily clinical practice upholding the Six 'C' core values of the nursing profession.

From a medical perspective concerning consent to disclosure of personal health information, the ethical debate has shifted to a new direction surrounding the European Court of Human Rights' (ECtHR) notion of European Convention on Human Rights (ECHR) Article 8, on the concept of a 'reasonable expectation' of privacy. Taylor and Wilson (2019) discuss its meaning relating to the disclosure of health data in current legal decisions concerning legal liability, arguing that implied consent is 'pushing the boundaries of claims that an individual has signalled their consent'. Considering that acceptance is more passive than consent, consent should then be considered more from the perspective of the patient than the medical professional; this favours the stance of respecting patient autonomy and dignity through 'reasonable expectation', thereby reducing the existing over-reliance upon implied consent (Taylor and Wilson, 2019).

Transferring ethical principles into good practices could suggest adopting the NHS Code of Practice model, which outlines the four main requirements that need to be met by those who hold recorded information concerning patients within their care (see Fig. 6.1).

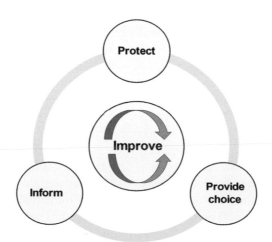

Fig. 6.1 Confidentiality model. (Adapted from Department of Health, 2003.)

This model provides a framework emphasising *protecting* the patient's information through secure storage, protocols and procedures of documentation and disclosure, *informing* patients of how their information is used, and ensuring that they are aware of how it is recorded and accessed. Based on the different needs and values of patients, providing *choice* allows them to decide whether their information can be disclosed and the ways in which it can be used (DH, 2003). To uphold these three requirements, healthcare managers and clinical staff should always seek better ways to protect confidential patient information, give advice and notify and provide choice for patients.

For more guidance on working safely with confidential patient information, the GMC (2017) publication *Confidentiality: good practice in handling patient information* provides a comprehensive framework for the legal and ethical duties and disclosures to support the direct care and protection of a patient and others. Although this guidance was written for medical professionals, it is of considerable relevance to professional nurses as well, and certainly of value for reference purposes, involving matters of information within routine clinical practice.

Access to Records – Statutory Provision

In accordance with the ECHR Article 8 'Rights to privacy', the main legislation regulating privacy and access to information is the General Data Protection Regulation (including DPA 2018) and the Freedom of Information Act 2000. This chapter presents an overview of the key aspects of this legislation as well as other related ones.

The General Data Protection Regulation (GDPR) was passed by the EU and took effect in May 2018, imposing obligations upon organisations who request and collect data from EU citizens (ICO, 2018). Its origins derive from the ECHR Article 8 'Right to Privacy'. In 1998, the European Data Protection Directive was passed to establish minimum data privacy and security standards; the GDPR is an update of this directive. If an organisation fails to comply with the GDPR, it can face financial penalties. Following the withdrawal of the UK from the EU in January 2021, the UK GDPR came into effect, and remained supplemented by the DPA 2018, whose prime purpose was to 'empower individuals to take control of their personal data and to support organisations with their lawful processing of personal data' (ICO, 2019). Organisations are regulated through such legislation by the Information Commissioner's Office (ICO), a UK independent body formed to uphold information rights in the public interest and data privacy for individuals by enforcing laws – namely the UK GDPR. According to Section 121 of the DPA, the ICO has produced a Code of Practice in conjunction with its regulation of communications, networking and data protection within and among organisations (ICO, 2020). As the data protection regulator, the ICO has the power to investigate organisations that have suffered data breaches, audit organisations for data storage and collection practices, and impose fines of up to £20 million for organisations that fail to prevent potential negligence due to a breach (ITPro, 2020).

Under Article 4 of the UK GDPR and DPA 2018, personal data is defined as any information relating to an individual (the data subject) who can be directly or indirectly identified by means of name, ID number, location/address (including web address), gender, ethnicity, religious or political beliefs. It includes factors specific to a person, such as physical, psychological, genetic, mental, economic, social or cultural identity. Healthcare provider services are responsible for the safekeeping of patient records under the GDPR. 'Adult health' records are kept for up to 8 years after the patient was last seen by the service; GP surgery records for 10 years after a patient has died; and mental health specific records for 20 years after a patient was last seen or discharged by psychiatric services or following their death.

The DPA applies to all people and in the context of healthcare, extends from a patient undergoing care to a person providing data about hospital services, for example, a complaint via the hospital's Patient Advice Liaison Service (PALS) team, or a public official connected with the local healthcare service. Such information does not have to be 'private', but information that is public knowledge or is about a person's professional life can be regarded as personal data. If an information is regarded as 'anonymous' but the person can still be identified by certain details if combined with other information, it is regarded as personal data. Data processing refers to any action performed on automated or manual data, including collecting, recording, organising, storing, using, transmitting and erasing. The requirements of GDPR Article 13 apply in this respect. An NHS Trust or a private hospital are examples of the persons who decide why and how personal data will be processed – the data controller and any services, employed, contracted or receiving data from the controller, are called data processors.

Therefore, a nurse is considered a data processor when handling patient information during their daily work activities. Certain types of personal data are defined by the GDPR as being more sensitive in nature and requiring a higher level of protection. Thus, the processing of data is prohibited if it reveals the following: race, ethnic origin, religious/philosophical beliefs, political opinions, trade union membership, genetic data, biometrics used for uniquely identifying an individual, health data and data concerning an individual's sexual orientation or sex life. Article 5 of the GDPR lists the six principles of personal data handling (Box 6.1):

BOX 6.1 ■ Principles of Personal Data Handling

Personal data shall be:
- Processed lawfully, fairly and in a transparent manner;
- Collected for specified, explicit and legitimate purposes;
- Adequate, relevant and limited to what is necessary;
- Accurate, and where necessary up to date;
- Stored for no longer than is necessary;
- Processed in a manner that ensures integrity and confidentiality.

Taken from ICO General Data Protection Regulations Article 5.

GDPR Articles 6 and 9 cover the lawful reasons for processing personal data. Nurses and healthcare professionals working in NHS organisations operate within the special category of health data, which includes the provision of health services that reveal information about a person's health status (Article 9). Under GDPR Article 4, a person's consent (an agreement) and explicit consent (where the person is given a clear verbal or written option to agree or disagree) is required for the lawful processing of personal data, and such consent must comprise a statement of action that is freely given, specific, informed and unambiguous. With the 'special category' of health data, GDPR Article 9 (2) requires explicit consent from the patient that allows for 'the processing of data for health purposes including medical diagnosis, the provision of health and social care or treatment or the management of health or social care systems'. GDPR Article 7 affirms that if the data subject (e.g. patient) has no genuine choice or is unable to withdraw consent without detriment, then consent cannot be regarded as freely given. To understand the patient's (as a data subject's) perspective, it is worth briefly outlining their rights under the GDPR, which data controllers must recognise and adhere to (Box 6.2).

BOX 6.2 ■ GDPR Rights for Patients (Data Subjects)

Transparency – The right to be informed clearly and privately.

Right to access held data – Within a time limit of one month.

Right to rectification – Data controllers must ensure that information is accurate, and respond to patients' request for rectification within one month.

Right to erasure – Applicable if the patient withdraws consent and there are no other legal grounds for processing, or where the patient objects and there is no overriding legitimate grounds; the data collected are used for commercial websites; and the personal data are no longer necessary for its original purpose of collection. The right is not available if the processing is for a task carried out for reasons of public interest, such as public health.

Right to restrict processing – Applicable when the accuracy of the data is contested, the processing is unlawful and the patient opposes erasure; the data controller no longer needs the data, but the patient requires them for legal claims purposes; the patient has objected until verification is made for legitimate reasons.

Right to data portability – Applicable when the patient has consented to the right to receive data in a commonly used machine-readable format that is automated.

Right to object to processing – On the grounds relating to the patient's situation concerning direct marketing purposes (an absolute right); for scientific or historical research (limited right); in the public interest and necessary for the controllers or third party's legitimate interests. The controller may continue processing the personal data if they can demonstrate compelling legitimate grounds which override the interest, rights and freedoms of the patient or for the establishment and exercise or defence of legal claims.

Right not to be subject to decision based on automated processing – Including profiling, which may include data concerning the patient's health or socio-economic status.

Adapted from the General Data Protection Regulations, chapter III.

Prior to the GDPR, a prominent case on common law right access to patient's health records was that of *R v Mid Glamorgan FHSA ex p Martin*. See Case study 6.2.

Notably, the only remaining provisions of the Access to Health Records Act 1990 are those involving the records of a deceased person, where such patients' personal representative or any person who may have a claim resulting from the death may apply for access to the relevant records.

When a claim is made on the grounds that the published material is defamatory and likely to cause serious harm to a person's reputation, particularly if the material is malicious and untrue, then the claim may be made upon the grounds of libel under the Defamation Act 2013. This was demonstrated in *Cornelius v De Taranto*, described in the following Case study 6.3.

Other cases that merit further study regarding breach of confidentiality are *Hunter v Mann*, concerning a dangerous driving offence and the duty of a doctor to disclose information where they are compelled to by law; *H (A Healthcare Worker) v Associated Newspapers Limited and N (A Health Authority)* concerning a healthcare worker diagnosed HIV-positive refusing (under Article 8) to disclose patient records to the Health Authority who required a 'look back' exercise to identify those who may have come into contact with the worker and were at risk of contracting HIV; and *Roberts v Nottinghamshire Healthcare NHS Trust*, where a patient at a high-security hospital sought access, under the DPA, to his psychological report but was refused.

The Freedom of Information Act 2000

The Freedom of Information Act 2000 (FOIA) created a statutory right of access to information relating to bodies that exercise functions of a public nature. These

CASE STUDY 6.2	R v Mid Glamorgan FHSA ex p Martin [1995] 1 All Er 356

Mr Martin had been a patient at a number of hospitals and sought from them all of his personal health and social care records. This was prior to the GDPR, and thus was subject to the Access to Health Records Act 1990 and the earlier Data Protection Act 1984. Hence, his claim had to be determined through common law. The hospitals concerned were willing to disclose the records to Mr Martin's legal advisers, but not directly to him. The judge dismissed his initial claim and declared it did not breach Article 8 of the ECHR. The Court of Appeal followed by rejecting Mr Martin's appeal in that the Health Authority owned the records, and thus can deny patient access if it was in the patient's best interests. Nonetheless, the judges made remarks that backed a patient's right to access their records; they said the assertion by a doctor of 'absolute ownership' of a patient's medical records was untenable and that such records were a duty requirement, to provide the medical history for future doctors as well as provide a record of diagnosis and treatment in case of future enquiry or dispute. Acting in Mr Martin's best interests, and taking the view that it was equally untenable for a patient to have the same absolute right of access to records, the court permitted Mr Martin's lawyers to use the records for the purposes of advising upon legal matters and for them to decide on what extent a disclosure from the records could be made to Mr Martin without causing him further psychological harm.

| CASE STUDY 6.3 | Cornelius v De Taranto (2001) EWCA Civ 1511 |

C brought a successful claim (under the then Defamation Act 1952) against forensic psychiatrist Dr de Taranto ('D') for both a breach of confidence and libel. C claimed that D, following an assessment of C, produced a written report containing a number of alleged defamatory statements, some of which were factually untrue and had been disclosed to her psychiatrist and GP without her implied consent. Consequently, it became part of C's NHS records. C had, in fact, refused to give consent to this disclosure and no record of consent was made in C's notes. The judge held that the test in determining the question of harm was to consider the statements from the perspective of less qualified persons rather than psychiatrists and qualified nurses, and that express consent should have been obtained, bearing in mind Article 8 of the ECHR. Damages were awarded for significant mental distress caused by the breach of confidence and the costs of obtaining the medical records.

bodies are public authorities, publicly owned companies and designated bodies performing public functions. The Freedom of Information (Scotland) Act was passed in 2002. As with the GDPR, this Act falls under the jurisdiction of the ICO, and NHS organisations are required to appoint a data protection officer whose overall responsibility is to keep a record of the data collected and its purpose, as well as the lawful reasoning for its processing. Over the past 30 years, 'digital revolution' has become integral to the running of the NHS and independent care providers, and information technology systems have to be planned and managed under the legislative frameworks of data protection and freedom of information. Thus, the Health and Social Care Act 2012 established the Health and Social Care Information Centre (HSCIC) as the principal provider of IT infrastructure and the management of data standards across healthcare organisations throughout the UK. This included faster and more secure access to clinical information. In July 2016, the HSCIC changed its name to NHS Digital.

The FOIA covers all recorded information including emails, telephone conversations, CCTV footage and land-mail correspondence. Through the FOIA, any person inside or outside the UK can request information from a public authority and be informed, in writing by that authority, whether it holds the information as specified in the request. If it does hold such information, then it needs to show how it will communicate such to the person making the request. The main principle behind the FOIA is that people have a right to know about the activities of public authorities (e.g. NHS, local authorities, government departments, police and state schools) in that such authorities spend tax-payers' money and make decisions that can significantly affect people's lives. Thus, access to information is an open way for these authorities to demonstrate accountability for their practices and enable the public to be better informed and make appropriate choices. Such transparency also enhances public confidence and trust. Disclosure of this information should be kept private only if there is good reason to do so and is permitted by the Act, with the authority justifying any refusal to issue the requested information. Response to a request must be provided within 20 working days, and all information requesters should be treated equally, with status in society or job title not allowing anyone privileged rights. The ICO has produced a guide to the complexities of FOIA requests (ICO, 2017); it is important to note that under Part 2 of the Act, there are exemptions under the broad categories of 'absolute' and 'qualified'. An absolute exemption means that there is no obligation to release the requested information, even though there may be other reasons outside the Act to do so; a qualified exemption implies that a public authority has to assess the balance of public interest for and against disclosing information, and justify any non-disclosure.

Absolute exemption would include:

- Information accessible to the applicant by other means if it is sourced from another eligible body or is already in a public information scheme.
- Court records.
- Parliamentary privilege – removes the duty to confirm or deny.
- Information provided in confidence, where the disclosure would resulted in an 'actionable breach' of confidence.
- Disclosure prohibited by other legislation – that is, another enactment.
- Personal information – falling within the scope of Data Protection.
- Prejudice to effective conduct of public affairs, which inhibits provision of advice and exchange of views for the purposes of deliberation.

Qualified exemption would include:

- Matters of defence or national security concerning the British Isles.
- International relations with other states and relations within the UK between governmental bodies.
- Investigations and proceedings conducted by the public authority with a view to bringing court proceedings or relating to information from confidential sources.
- Health and safety concerns, endangering the physical or mental health of an individual.
- Legal professional privilege.
- Formulation of government policy, including ministerial communications and private office functions.
- Communications with Her Majesty and Royal Family.

If a freedom of information request is made by a patient who is the data subject and wants access to personal information, then this should be refused and treated accordingly as a data protection subject access request via the GDPR. An organisation is not obliged to confirm or deny as to whether they hold the personal information if this would disclose personal data relating to the requester. The 2007 case of *Bluck v Information Commissioner and another* illustrates the FOIA's absolute exemption from disclosure, when a hospital owes a duty of confidence to a deceased person which, if breached, could be actionable by the next of kin following the patient's death. When considering sharing information for auditing, teaching or research purposes, such information is usually anonymised through the removal of all clear identifiers, such as names, addresses, NHS number and date of birth, thus no longer rendering it confidential. The case of *R v Department of Health ex parte Source Informatics Ltd* provides a good illustration of the threshold concerning anonymised patient information.

Other Relevant Legislation

The <u>Access to Medical Reports Act 1988</u> gives patients the right to view their medical reports for employment or insurance purposes, written by a medical practitioner whom they usually see in a normal doctor-patient capacity. This includes reports from a GP, occupational health doctor and/or a specialist who has provided care. This right can be exercised before or after the report is sent and the patient must be afforded the opportunity within 21 days to view the report and be allowed to correct any errors or raise any disagreement with the matters of fact recorded. Thus, the patient has the right to withdraw their consent for the release of the report. There is an exemption from the patient accessing the report, when the medical practitioner opines that the disclosure would likely cause serious mental or physical harm to the patient or where the identity of another person would be made known, unless they were a healthcare professional or a person who had consented to the disclosure.

The <u>Human Fertilisation and Embryology Act 1990 (UK) Section 33A</u> protects the confidentiality of information kept by clinics and the Human Fertilisation and Embryology Authority. Access to or disclosure of information can only be done under specific circumstances set out in the Act. It is an offence to disclose information that identifies the patient in other circumstances without the patient's prior consent.

The <u>National Health Service (Venereal Diseases) Regulations 1974 (Wales) and the NHS Trusts and Primary Care Trusts (Sexually Transmitted Diseases) Directions 2000 (England)</u> stipulate that any information that makes it possible to identify an individual who is examined or treated for a sexually transmitted disease shall not be disclosed, other than to a medical practitioner linked to the treatment of the individual relating to the disease or for the prevention of the spread of the disease.

The <u>Health and Social Care (Safety and Quality) Act 2015 (England)</u> is intended to improve the safety and quality of health and social care. The Act proposed new rules relating to professional regulation, information sharing across organisations and avoidable harm to patients. The Act established the former HSCIC (now NHS Digital) to set information standards for commissioners and providers to appropriately share information supporting people's direct care in England. In making an overarching objective of public protection, the Act gave the Professional Standards Authority for Health and Social Care further directives to promote more effective self-regulation and cooperation between health and care regulators (e.g. the NMC) and corresponding bodies.

<u>Section 251 of the NHS Act 2006 (England and Wales)</u> allows the Secretary of State for Health to make regulations that set aside the common law duty of confidentiality for defined medical purposes. That is, the person responsible for information, within regulatory requirements, can disclose confidential patient information without their consent to an applicant without breaching the duty of confidentiality. This must comply with the relevant obligations of the DPA 1998 and Human Rights Act (HRA) 1998. The <u>Health Service (Control of Patient Information) Regulations 2002</u> enables this power with reference to 'Section 251 support or approval' which gives

authority of the regulations. Such powers can only be used where it is not practical to obtain consent and where anonymised information cannot be used; information disclosed solely or principally for the direct care of individual patients is not permitted.

The Police and Criminal Evidence Act 1984, under Sections 9, 12 and 14, gives police the powers to take medical records, human tissue or tissue fluid for the purpose of diagnosis or medical treatment which a person holds in confidence. This includes personal records which a person 'has acquired or created in course of any trade, business or profession…' or personal records or documents concerning an individual (including deceased) relating to their health, including '…counselling or assistance given or to be given to him for the purposes of his personal welfare, by any voluntary organisation…'. A county court judge can make an order that a person who appears to be in possession of the specified material, which is an item other than that subject to legal privilege and excluded material, produce it to a police officer to access and be taken away.

The Gender Recognition Act 2004 (UK) Section 22 is designed to protect the privacy rights of transsexual people under Article 8 of the ECHR by criminalising the disclosure of information, where it is an offence to disclose protected information to any other person when that information is acquired in an official capacity. In this instance, 'protected information' is that concerning a person's application for gender recognition and their gender history after they have changed their gender. This part of the Act also provides gives justifiable exceptions for disclosure to be considered. These are detailed within the Gender Recognition (Disclosure of Information) (England, Wales and Northern Ireland) Order 2005 and The Gender Recognition (Disclosure of Information) (Scotland) Order 2005.

The Public Interest Disclosure Act 1998 authorises 'qualified disclosures', which are breaches in confidence that are permitted if an organisation's employee believes there is criminal activity, failure to comply with an obligation of the law, a miscarriage of justice or risk of an individual's health and safety. Injustice may be considered a suitable cause for a breach, and those who report wrongful or illegal activity, 'whistle-blowers', are offered protection through the Act.

The Influence of 'Caldicott'

In December 1997, the UK government review of Patient Identifiable Information set out principles for determining the use of confidential information, and made 26 recommendations concerning aspects such as access to electronic care records, information sharing (or opting out) among an individual's care team and breaches of information governance (DH, 1997). The review committee was chaired by Dame Fiona Caldicott, who had a professional background as a Consultant Psychiatrist, and since 2018, has been the statutory National Data Guardian (NDG) for Health and Social Care. The other central element of the review was the recommendation that every healthcare organisation nominate a senior person to act as a 'guardian' responsible for safeguarding the confidentiality of patient information and promoting the principles set out in the review recommendations. This 'guardian' was designated to be part of the organisation's senior management team with strategic and governance responsibilities, providing leadership and informed guidance through the complex process of confidentiality and information sharing. Ultimately, this guardian was responsible for the arrangements within the organisation that ensured that the confidential information (e.g. medical records) of service users be utilised in a legal, ethical and appropriate manner. Since 1999, NHS organisations have been required to have a Caldicott Guardian (HSC 1999/012), as have Local Authority Social services in England since 2002 (HSC 2002/003 LAC (2002)2). Although a mandatory requirement, it was left to the individual organisations to determine how their 'guardians' would operate. The National Data Guardian for Health and Social Care was formed as an independent body serving to advise as a non-regulatory 'point of contact' for over 1800 Caldicott Guardians (NDG, 2020).

The original principles were revised through a later review (DH, 2013), often referred to as 'Caldicott 2'. This was reviewed again following a consultation in 2019 (NDG, 2020), which resulted in a further revision, leading to the current existence of the eight principles outlined in Box 6.3.

The principles are proposed to apply to all data collected for the provision of health and social care services in which service users (e.g. patients) can be identified, and where they expect that their data will be secure and private; for example, particulars about diagnosis, treatment, names and addresses. Service users should be regarded as partners with their care and associated healthcare records. As Alderson (2014) notes, it is probable that most NHS patients have not given much thought to the extent to which their information is shared over the years, whether in anonymised or identifiable form; they may have believed that 'the issue was too complex to attempt to explain to patients proactively' (Alderson, 2014). It is important for nurses to be aware that just as there are patients who are well aware of their rights concerning their personal data, so too are there patients who merely assume that their healthcare providers may share and use information relating to their

---

BOX 6.3 ■ The Caldicott Principles

- Justify the purposes for using confidential information
- Use confidential information only when it is necessary
- Use the minimum necessary information
- Access to confidential information should be on a strict need-to-know basis
- Everyone with access to confidential information should be aware of their responsibilities
- Comply with the law
- The duty to share information for individual care is as important as the duty to protect patient confidentiality
- Inform patients and service users about how their confidential information is used

Taken from United Kingdom Caldicott Guardian Council, 2020 (revised). A manual for Caldicott guardians. Available at: https://www.ukcgc.uk/manual/contents.

care, sometimes in ways that may go beyond the law. Therefore, the nurse has some responsibility in protecting the patient's rights in a transparent manner that informs the patient of them and raising such matters within the provider organisation.

References

Alderson, C, 2014. Information governance in the NHS: Caldicott 2 and beyond. Clinical Risk 19 (6), 115–119.

Avery, G, 2013. Law and ethics in nursing and healthcare: an introduction. Sage Publications, London.

Beauchamp, T, Childress, J, 2019. Principles of biomedical ethics, 8th ed. Oxford University Press, New York.

Department of Health, 1997. The Caldicott Committee: report on the review of patient-identifiable information. Available at: https://static.ukcgc.org.uk/docs/caldicott1.pdf.

Department of Health, 2003. Confidentiality: code of practice. Crown Copyright.

Department of Health, 2010. Confidentiality: NHS code of practice. Supplementary guidance: public interest disclosures. Available at: http://www.dh.gov.uk/publications.

Department of Health, 2013. Information: to share or not to share. Government response to the Caldicott review, London.

General Medical Council, 2017. Confidentiality: good practice in handling patient information. Available at: https://www.gmc-uk.org/.

Information Commissioner's Office, 2017. The guide to freedom of information. Available at: https://ico.org.uk/media/for-organisations/guide-to-freedom-of-information-4-9.pdf.

Information Commissioner's Office, 2018. Guide to the General Data Protection Regulation. Available at: https://www.gov.uk/government/publications/guide-to-the-general-data-protection-regulation.

Information Commissioner's Office, 2019. An overview of the Data Protection Act 2018 (version 2). Available at: https://ico.org.uk/media/for-organisations/documents/2614158/ico-introduction-to-data-protection-bill.pdf.

Information Commissioner's Office, 2020. Data sharing code of practice. Available at: https://ico.org.uk/for-organisations/guide-to-data-protection/ico-codes-of-practice/data-sharing-a-code-of-practice/.

ITPro (2020). What is the Information Commissioner's Office? Available at: https://www.itpro.co.uk/information-commissioner/31751/what-is-the-information-commissioner-s-office-ico.

Messer, NG, 2004. Professional-patient relationships and informed consent. Post-graduate. Medical Journal 80, 277–283.

National Data Guardian, 2020. The National Data Guardian's response to the consultation on the Caldicott principles and Caldicott guardians. Available at: https://www.gov.uk/government/organisations/national-data-guardian.

Robinson, R, Doody, O, 2021. Nursing and healthcare ethics. Elsevier Health Sciences, Oxford.

Taylor, MJ, Wilson, J, 2019. Reasonable expectations of privacy and disclosure of health data. Medical Law Review 27 (3), 432–460.

United Kingdom Caldicott Guardian Council, 2020 (revised). A manual for Caldicott guardians. Available at: https://www.ukcgc.uk/manual/contents.

Wheeler, H, 2012. Law, ethics and professional issues for nursing: a reflective and portfolio-building approach. Routledge Taylor & Francis, London.

CASES

Bluck v Information Commissioner and another (2007) 98 BMLR 1
Cornelius v de Taranto [2001] EWCA Civ 1511
H (A Healthcare Worker) v Associated Newspapers Limited and N (A Health Authority) [2002] Lloyd's Rep Med 210 CA
Hunter v Mann [1974] QB 767
Palmer v Tees Health Authority [1999] EWCA Civ 1533
Public Health (Infectious Disease) Regulations 1988
R v Department of Health ex parte Source Informatics Ltd [2000] 1 All Er 786
Roberts v Nottinghamshire Healthcare NHS Trust [2008] EWHC (QB)
Tarasoff v Regents of the University of California [1976] 17 Cal 3d 425.
W v Egdell [1990] 2 WLR 471
Woolgar v Chief Constable of Sussex Police [2000] 1 WLR 25

STATUTE

Abortion Regulations 1991
Access to Medical Reports Act 1988
Births and Deaths Registration Act 1953
Coroners and Justice Act 2009
Data Protection Act 1998
Defamation Act 2013
Freedom of Information Act 2000
Gender Recognition Act 2004 (UK) Section 22
Gender Recognition (Disclosure of Information) (England, Wales and Northern Ireland) Order 2005
Gender Recognition (Disclosure of Information) (Scotland) Order 2005.
General Data Protection Regulation (including Data Protection Act 2018)
Health Service (Control of Patient Information) Regulations 2002
Health and Social Care Act 2012
Health and Social Care (Safety and Quality) Act 2015 (England)
Human Fertilisation and Embryology Act 1990 (UK) Section 33A
Misuse of Drugs Act 1971
Motor Vehicles (Driving Licenses) Regulations 1999
National Health Service (Venereal Diseases) Regulations 1974 (Wales)
NHS Trusts and Primary Care Trusts (Sexually Transmitted Diseases) Directions 2000 (England)
NHS Act 2006 (England and Wales) Section 251
Police and Criminal Evidence Act 1984
Prevention of Terrorism Act 2005
Public Health (Infectious Disease) Regulations 1988
Public Interest Disclosure Act 1998
Road Traffic Act 1988

Defensible Documentation

Introduction

All nurses are responsible for managing patient-care documents in accordance with the law and for complying with the Caldicott Principles and the standards set out by the Nursing and Midwifery Council (NMC). Record-keeping is a central aspect of nurses' duties; accordingly, the patient care and clinical interventions should be recorded as per clear, accurate and unambiguous standards. Standard 10 of the NMC Code (2018) states that a nurse should 'keep clear and accurate records relevant to your practice', although this is not limited to patient records. The *Oxford English Dictionary, (2011)* defines *documentation* as 'the accumulation… dissemination of information; material collected…; the collection of documents relating to a process or event…'; it defines *record* as '…a piece of evidence or information constituting an account of something that has occurred…'. The Data Protection Act 2018 defines 'health record' as '…a record which consists of data concerning health and has been made by or on behalf of a health professional in connection with the diagnosis, care or treatments of the individual to whom the data relates' (NHSX, 2021). Guidance and a framework for practice has been provided by the NHS – *A guide to the management of health and care records* (NHSX, 2021).

Defensible Health Records

The main purpose of keeping nursing records is to maintain an account of the care and treatment received by a patient and to monitor the patient's progress in a quantifiable manner. Defensible records are those that can justify a nurse's care and treatment interventions. If such records are presented as evidence in a court, considerable reliance may be placed upon them. As Griffith and Dowie (2019) explain… 'Any weaknesses in record keeping will hamper the professional when it comes to giving evidence in court and will render them vulnerable in cross-examination, especially when there has been a considerable delay between the events recorded and the court hearing'. Such records include patient clinical notes, e-mails and phone texts, laboratory or x-ray reports, printouts from monitoring equipment, incident reports and statements, recordings of telephone or online 'conference' calls and letters between professionals, both internal to the organisation and external from other agencies or care providers. Fundamentally, when a patient interacts with a healthcare professional, documentation can serve as a record of what has occurred, underscoring that record-keeping is an integral part of healthcare practice. Effective record-keeping should assist in maintaining the continuity of care and promote an overall high standard of care; it can also be an indicator of a skilled nurse. Furthermore, any notes or records taken in the course of a nurse's duties are potentially legal documents that can be subpoenaed to court. Thus, nurses should always be mindful in ensuring that their clinical records are robust enough to present a true and detailed picture such that it defends their professional decision-making and actions.

Major case reviews and public enquiries where the quality of clinical records were criticised include the *University Hospitals of Morecambe Bay NHS Foundation Trust* [Care Quality Commission (CQC, 2012)]; *Mid Staffordshire NHS Foundation Trust Inquiry* (2010) and the *Liverpool Care Pathway* (Neuberger, 2013). Therefore, healthcare professionals must be accountable for safe and effective record-keeping as part of their duty of care, and must bear in mind that this is an integral aspect of the requirements directed by their regulatory body.

Common Faults in Record-Keeping

Although effective record-keeping strengthens nurses' accountability, many nurses have experienced problems identified with poor record-keeping practice. A comprehensive list of common faults with nursing records presented by Griffith and Dowie (2019) constitutes a useful reference:

- Illegible handwriting
- Ambiguous abbreviations
- Omission of time of events and inaccuracies of dates
- Use of 'tippex' to cover-up errors
- Lack of staff signature
- Absence of key clinical information
- Delay, sometimes of more than 24 hours, before records are completed
- Inaccuracy of patient's name, address and date of birth
- Unprofessional terminology (e.g. lay-jargon)
- Opinion mixed with facts and subjective comments
- Completed by another person who has not undertaken the care

The Legal Perspective

The fundamental standards for healthcare record management are provided by Regulation 17 (2) (c) of the Health and Social Care Act 2008 (Regulated Activities) Regulations 2014. It states that a care provider should 'maintain securely an accurate, complete and contemporaneous record in respect of each service user, including a record of the care and treatment provided to the service user and of decisions taken in relation to the care and treatment provided' (CQC, 2021). Any notes or records (typed or handwritten) made in the course of a nurse's duties are a potential legal document and can be subpoenaed to court as part of evidence gathering for a case. As such documentation may be reviewed and scrutinised by lawyers and expert witnesses, its timeliness, accuracy, completeness, legibility and relevance are essential in determining the facts of a case. In 2019–2020, proven allegations of poor record-keeping formed 16% of the cases in the top three categories dealt with by the NMC regulatory processes (NMC, 2020).

Cases may come to court years after an event has occurred, and the nurse may well find that their recollection of events is not very clear due to the passage of time. Accurate documentation can provide vital evidence to demonstrate the nurses' actions, enabling them to relate incidents as precisely as possible. Conversely, the circumstances of events in question may be fresh in the memory of a patient or their relatives and carers, so any vagueness, unsubstantiated detail or judgemental views may be viewed as a lack of professional credibility in a court. Griffith (2007) emphasises that cases can be won or lost on the strength of records and comments: '…in litigation, the outcome is not based on truth but proof. If it is not in the notes, it can be difficult to prove it happened'. Case study 7.1 outlines a notable case that highlights the importance of accurate, contemporaneous recording of clinical events.

Other notable cases concerning the importance of documentation include *Prendergast v Sam and Dee*, where an illegible prescription resulted in the patient being given the wrong drug and harmed as a consequence; *McLennan v Newcastle HA*, concerning the recording of a patient being told of the risks of a surgical procedure; *Kent v Griffiths & Others*, concerning contemporaneous falsification of emergency ambulance records; and *FE (Represented by his litigation friend PE) v St George's*

CASE STUDY 7.1	Saunders v Leeds Western HA [1993] 4 Med LR 355

A four-year-old girl suffered a cardiac arrest that lasted 40 minutes during an arthroplasty operation, and hypoxia resulted in her suffering permanent brain damage, blindness and paraplegia. Even though the theatre staff argued that the girl's pulse had stopped suddenly and the cardiac arrest was due to a hidden air embolism blocking a major artery, there was no evidence in the records to indicate this, and it was thus deemed implausible. This case was an example of *Res ipsa loquitur*, where the plaintiff cannot identify the precise nature of the harm, but negligence can be inferred. The court was of the opinion that a fit four-year-old would not normally suffer cardiac arrest if the correct anaesthesia protocols were followed. The defendants were held liable.

University Hospitals NHS Trust, concerning inadequate record-keeping, including poor identification of who had made entries.

Effective Record-Keeping

In emphasising that recording care is not distinct from the actual provision of care, Beach and Oates (2014) state that sufficient time should be allocated for documentation. However, though nurses may be aware of the principles of good record-keeping, they may struggle to put these principles into practice. Clinical records should be clear, unambiguous, and legible and aid the continuity of care by providing an effective method of communication. Handwritten records should be in black ink, as they may need to be photocopied in future for legal purposes or for use in an inquiry, as well as to avoid illegible signatures requiring the addition of the name and position of the nurse making the entry. Whether in handwritten or electronic format, it is important to use plain language, avoid jargon, be objective in presentation and only use abbreviations as designated and recognised by the healthcare provider organisation.

Records should be factual and not opinion-based. Nurses must use their professional judgement in considering what to record, in addition to taking into account the other professionals involved in the patient's care. They should always attribute entries to themselves, never make entries on behalf of another health worker, and use quotation marks, if necessary, to record what exactly was spoken. On occasions, nurses may need to countersign an entry made by an unregistered member of staff or student nurse. If an error or alteration is made within the record-keeping process, the error must be struck through with a line with the initials of the person and date of making the correction is required; completely obliterating the error is unacceptable. Electronic records often have an addendum where the correction can be detailed.

Clinical records also need to be accurate and contemporaneous in their presentation; thus, all entries in a patient's records should be made as soon as possible after an intervention or a relevant event in the patient's treatment and care. Any lapse in time between the intervention/event and the recording should be identifiable by the date and time of the recording being made and of the intervention/event. Daily records should include all nursing assessments, interventions and follow-up care with the patient's response to care and treatment, in addition to detailing any deterioration in the patient's health and identified risks. This should include the measures the nurse has taken to address any risk factors or deterioration (and improvement) in the patient's health; it is also good practice to give a reasoned rationale for any decision recorded about a patient's care. In making sure that other professionals who access the patient records have relevant and accurate information, nurses must recognise that clinical record-keeping is a continual, ongoing process where alongside each entry is information regarding date, time, name and job title of the nurse. However, in a complex, busy clinical environment, consistently maintaining effective record-keeping can be challenging. To this end, Doran's (1981) widespread SMART (Specific Measurable Achievable Relative and Timely objectives) framework can prove useful when entering and reviewing records. Furthermore, Brook's (2021) paper provides a detailed procedure for record-keeping, providing a sound aide-memoire framework for assisting the nurse in making safe and effective record entries when accounting for patient care and nursing interventions.

When not in use, all patient records should be stored securely, either in key-locked storage for paper documents and as encrypted and password protected for electronic documents. The safekeeping of such records should be in line with Caldicott requirements, the provider organisation's own policy and protocols, and the duty requirements of the Public Records Act 1958 (Section 3).

The period of time for retention of health records varies depending upon the type of record. Table 7.1 gives examples of the most common types of health care records and their retention time limits.

Electronic Health Records

The advancement of Information Technology has resulted in developments in the recording and storage of documentation relating to treatment and care within provider services. Electronic health records (EHRs) are fast becoming the norm throughout the UK. EHRs have greatly enhanced multi-professional communication between primary and secondary services and have resolved problems that can arise from manual paper records, such as omissions of key data and illegible handwriting. However, even with EHRs, the principles of effective record-keeping still apply in the same way as with manual records, and fall under the regulatory scrutiny of the General Data Protection Regulation (GDPR) and Data Processing Agreement (DPA). Other benefits of EHRs include the capability of healthcare professionals to gain quick access to an application at any time for key information, such as a patient's history or recent diagnostic tests, for example, X-rays. These records can also assist the nurse in sending and receiving information between departments and care providers to support coordinated care, and enable them to find or request information regarding a patient, particularly during unplanned care, such as the accident and emergency department. An illustration of such improved access to information is provided by the NHS Summary Care Record (SCR), which was introduced throughout primary care in 2010 and provides the accessible, secure storage of key patient information from General Practice surgeries including the patient's name, address, date of birth, NHS number, prescribed medication and allergies (NHS Digital, 2020).

Despite technological advancements, the ethical principle of respecting personal autonomy still includes privacy and an individual's control over their personal information. Nevertheless, privacy breaches do occur. Neame (2014) outlines the five principle sources of privacy breaches within electronic health records:

- Inadequate identification and authentication of those accessing private records.
- Ready accessibility of stored information; unrestricted access and read/write privileges available to more users than necessary. Includes inadequate logging of user activity and abuse of access rights.

TABLE 7.1 ■ Most Common Types of Health Care Records and Their Retention Time Limits

Type of Record	Legal Time Limit
General Practitioner records	For the life of the patient and up until 10 years after the patient's death
Adult health records	Eight years
Adult social care records	Eight years
Patient complaint files	Ten years
Serious incidents requiring investigation	Twenty years
Incidents – not serious	Ten years
Advanced medical therapy	Thirty years
Clinical Trials Master file authorised under EU regulation 536/2014	Twenty-five years
Post-mortem records	Ten years
NHS medicals for adoption records	Eight years or 25th birthday
Cause of death certificate	Two years
Mortuary records of deceased persons	Ten years
Register of birth	Two years
Register of death	Two years
Local authority adoption register	Hundred years
Transplantation records	Thirty years
Operating theatre records	Ten years
Clinical diaries	Two years
Pharmacy prescription records	Two years
Obstetrics, maternity, antenatal and postnatal records	Twenty-five years
Prison health records	Ten years
Contraception/sexual health/family planning/genito-urinary medicine	Eight to ten years
Cancer/oncology records	Thirty years or eight years after death
General dental services records	Eight years
Children's records (including midwifery, health visiting and school nursing)	Up to 25th birthday or 26th birthday if patient was 17 when treatment ended
Mental health records, including Psychology services	Twenty years or eight years after death
Secure mental health units	Twenty years or longer if justified and permitted
Long-term illness or illness that may re-occur	Thirty years or eight years after death

- Inappropriate disclosure without authorisation from the patient, such as through other portable devices (e.g. USB sticks; notebooks) that are inadequately secured.
- Statutory reporting requirements, primary legislation and departmental directives, which require in-confidence disclosures of personal information.
- Poor security, including protection from external 'hackers' and malware, but also, allowing users to access records externally and remotely after by-passing security controls.

Regarding users being given information system access privileges, Neame (2014) raises the concern that users are '…not made explicitly aware of their responsibilities or limits, nor of the penalties for abuses'. Therefore, it is essential that nurses understand their legal and ethical responsibilities of recording and using EHRs. During the course of day-to-day clinical duties, nurses with limited awareness may develop incorrect practices, such as 'borrowing' a colleague's *userID*, and their electronic record usage may be incompatible with GDPR requirements. In adhering to good practice and maintaining legally defensible documentation, the Information Commissioner's Office (ICO) provides guidance for operating within the scope of the UK GDPR's, and, in particular, Article 5 (1) (f), which details the 'Security Principle' concerning its regulatory function.

To assist the nurse in practising safely when accessing EHRs, the author has designed a seven-point checklist (Box 7.1) of key principles to help ensure nurses' working awareness of practising safely and ethically.

BOX 7.1 ■ Responsibilities for Self-Managing Electronic Patient Records: A Checklist for Nurses

- That you are authorised to access the e-Records and identifiable by a unique User ID, being aware that all your actions (including timings) will leave a 'footprint' that can be tracked for the purposes of audit, monitoring and investigation.
- That you have a clear understanding of your privileges and responsibilities, and can self-regulate to avoid misuse and abuse of the e-Records system.
- That you monitor access to the e-Records system and help prevent unauthorised users from accessing records and functions.
- That when exporting data from the e-Records system, you have gained the appropriate authorisation as per your organisation's policy, and that you have exported the minimum data required for its purpose. Security should be ensured through encrypted access to the data and by certification that the recipient's organisational security provisions meet approval.
- That you dispose of personal health information such that it cannot be recovered from the deleted media or backup copies.
- That your provider organisation has access to IT staff and that such staff are overseen so that they do not view patient information, which is not required within their role.
- That you fully understand the 'Caldicott principles' and how to access the organisation's Caldicott Guardian for advice.

To conclude, all too often, clinical record-keeping is viewed as a necessary chore during a nurse's daily duties. However, nursing records contribute to the documentary evidence-base about the care and treatment each patient receives, principally that of progress notes, assessments, care plans and multi-disciplinary communications. Effective nursing care records are not only essential nursing tools that enable continuity of care and safe decision-making, but are also valuable in providing sound evidence of the care provided, where, if the quality of the care is called into doubt, then those nursing records can provide documentation essential to any investigation or review. From a governance perspective, good practice in record-keeping and documentation handling gives an indication that care meets the set standards of quality and safety expected by professional regulators, and fulfils the contractual requirements set by healthcare commissioners.

References

Beach, J, Oates, J, 2014. Maintaining best practice in record-keeping and documentation. Nursing Standard 28 (36), 45–50.

Brooks, N, 2021. How to undertake effective record-keeping and documentation. Nursing Standard 36 (4), 31–33.

Care Quality Commission, 2012. Investigation report: University Hospitals of Morecambe Bay NHS Foundation Trust. CQC, London.

Care Quality Commission, 2021. Regulation 17: Good governance. Available at: https://www.cqc.org.uk/guidance-providers/regulations-enforcement/regulation-17-good-governance#guidance.

Doran, GT, 1981. There's a S.M.A.R.T. way to write management's goals and objectives. Management Review 70 (11), 35–36.

Griffith, R, 2007. The importance of earnest record keeping. Nurse Prescribing 5 (8), 363–366.

Griffith, R, Dowie, I, 2019. Dimond's legal aspects of nursing, 8th ed. Pearson Education Ltd, London.

Nursing and Midwifery Council, 2018. The Code: professional standards of practice and behaviour for nurses, midwives and nursing associates.

Nursing and Midwifery Council, 2020. Annual fitness to practise report, 2019–2020. Available at: https://www.nmc.org.uk/globalassets/sitedocuments/annual_reports_and_accounts/ftpanelreports/2019-2020.

Mid Staffordshire NHS Foundation Trust Inquiry, 2010. Independent inquiry into care provided by Mid Staffordshire NHS Foundation Trust: January 2005–March 2009, vol. 1. The Stationery Office, London.

Neame, RLB, 2014. Privacy protection for personal health information and shared care records. Informatics in Primary Care 21 (2), 84–91.

Neuberger, J, 2013. More care, less pathway: independent review of the Liverpool care pathway. Available at: https://www.gov.uk/government/publications/review-of-liverpool-care-pathway-for-dying-patients.

NHS Digital, 2020. Summary care records (SCR). Available at: https://digital.nhs.uk/services/summary-care-records-scr.

NHSX, 2021. Records management code of practice 2021: A guide to the management of health and care records. Available at: http://www.nhsx.nhs.uk/information-governance/guidance/records-management-code/.

Oxford Dictionaries, 2011. Concise Oxford English dictionary, 12th ed. Oxford University Press, Oxford.

CASES

FE (Represented by his litigation friend PE) v St George's University Hospitals NHS Trust [2016] EWHC 553 (QB)
Kent v Griffiths & Others [2001] QB 36
McLennan v Newcastle HA [1992] 3 Med LR 215
Prendergast v Sam and Dee [1989] 1 Med LR 36
Saunders v Leeds Western HA [1993] 4 Med LR 355

STATUTES

Data Protection Act 2018
Health and Social Care Act 2008 (Regulated Activities) Regulations 2014
Public Records Act 1958

Consent and Mental Capacity

KEY TERMS

Capacity

Consent

Mental Capacity Act

Best Interests

Advance decisions

Independent Mental Capacity
Advocate

Medical paternalism

Introduction

The key legal principles of the Nursing and Midwifery Council (NMC) Code of Practice (Part 4) provide that a nurse should not only 'balance the need to act in the best interests of people at all times... respect a person's right to accept or refuse treatment' and to 'keep to all relevant laws about mental capacity...' but also 'make sure that the rights of those who lack capacity are still at the centre of the decision-making process' (NMC, 2018). In knowing that patients must provide informed consent before receiving any form of care or treatment, nurses must be fully aware of the legal basis underpinning such consent. It is important that they have a complete understanding of what a person 'without capacity to consent' implies. Such knowledge is required in making decisions that are in the patient's best interests, and to necessitate consideration within daily clinical decision-making, generally made on the basis of both intuitive and analytical judgement.

Consent and Capacity

Consent is an agreement by choice by one who has the freedom and capacity to make that choice (Oxford Dictionary of Law, 2018). In healthcare, informed consent is based on the moral and legal foundation of patient autonomy, in that patients have a basic legal and ethical right to decide what happens to their bodies. In the context of medicine, consent refers to the rights of patients to decide what clinical care they receive; it is the duty of doctors to ensure that patients give their permission prior to any examination or intervention. Capacity for self-determination is the legal recognition of a person's autonomy, and is a status granted by law of one person by another, such as in a doctor-patient relationship. Mental capacity refers to the ability to make a decision, and a lack of capacity is where 'a person lacks capacity in relation to a matter if at the material time he is unable to make a decision for himself in relation to the matter because of an impairment of, or a disturbance in the functioning of, the mind or brain' [Mental Capacity Act (MCA, 2005), Section 2:1]. The Mental Capacity Act (hereafter, the Act) provides the legal framework for acting and making decisions on behalf of individuals who lack the capacity to make specific decisions about themselves. Therefore, it is essential for nurses to be aware of their duty of care obligations to comply with the law on consent, respect patient autonomy and understand the need to comply with the 'Act' when assessing a patient's capacity; they must also know how to work with patients who are deemed incapacitated.

Much of the clinical treatment a patient receives involves some degree of physical touching of the patient by the healthcare professional. An invasive treatment, such as a surgical operation, is an example where 'touch' is necessary. Any unauthorised touching of a patient could constitute the crime of battery (if it is intentional) and the tort of trespass – deliberately avoiding the patient's consent. To act lawfully when touching a patient, the healthcare professional would require a defence of what Herring (2018) describes as a 'legal flak jacket', which was raised in the Court of Appeal decision in *Re W (a minor: medical treatment);* the three 'flak jackets' available are:

- The consent of the patient
- The consent of another person who is authorized to consent on the behalf of the patient; for example, the consent of a parent for the treatment of a child
- A specific defence in common law or statute, for example, the defence of necessity

A later Court of Appeal decision in *R (Burke) v GMC* reinforced the importance of the patient's right to refuse treatment, emphasising that 'where a competent patient makes it clear that he does not wish to receive treatment which is, objectively, in his medical best interests, it is unlawful for doctors to administer that treatment. Personal autonomy or the right of self-determination prevails'. However, as Herring (2018) notes, autonomy and self-determination do not entitle the patient to demand a particular medical treatment. When, then, does trespass lead to what may be deemed a breach of duty of care where reasonable, foreseeable damage has resulted for a claimant to seek damages on the grounds of negligence? A defence to a trespass claim is real if consent has been obtained from a patient who has been given information as to the broad risks associated with a medical procedure. Additionally, consent based on the knowledge not only of those broad risks but also more comprehensive knowledge, such as a more detailed discussion of such risks, is necessary for a defence in a claim in negligence. The slight distinction between the defences of negligence and trespass was considered in *Chatterton v Gerson* (Case study 8.1).

CASE STUDY 8.1	Chatterton v Gerson [1981] 1 All ER 257

The claimant (Mrs Chatterton) suffered severe pain due to a post-surgical scar in her groin. The defendant (Dr Gerson – a specialist doctor in pain treatment) advised surgery, but informed the claimant that there was a risk of numbness and temporary muscle weakness. A sensory nerve block operation was performed but it only provided temporary relief and caused numbness in the claimant's leg; further surgery was undertaken, but on that occasion, the defendant failed to warn the claimant that she might experience numbness or muscle weakness; he assumed that the claimant was aware of these after the first operation. The claimant completely lost sensation in her right leg and the pain worsened, which led her to suing the defendant for negligence and battery. The High Court ruled in favour of the defendant, deciding that he had fulfilled his duty of care by giving sufficient information and gaining valid consent from the claimant. For the purpose of the tort of battery, the operation's nature and purpose had been explained in 'broad terms', and consent was only valid if the claimant had been informed of the broad nature of the defendant's actions and not every risk associated with such actions.

The more recent case of *Montgomery v Lanarkshire Health Board* provides better insight into the respect of this duty, where patients, as consumers, can consider choices and exercise their rights to decide rather being passive recipients of the treatment by the medical professional. Nurses must ensure that information is presented to the patient in an understandable way (e.g. by avoiding medical jargon). As *Montgomery* states, the patient should be 'given time and space as far as is reasonably practicable' to weigh the options before deciding on a treatment option. The decision-making process and information shared should be carefully recorded by the nurse (Taylor, 2018). *Montgomery* is discussed later in this chapter (Case study 8.3).

Mode and Conditions for Valid Consent

There is no legal distinction between written and verbal consent; however, in some cases, such as a major surgery, it is customary to ask a patient to sign a consent form, as this can indicate precisely what the patient has been told and what they have consented to. A medical practitioner should obtain consent for each medical procedure and not assume that because the patient has consented to past procedures, they will naturally consent to further procedures. Consent can be either expressed or implied. Implied consent implies that the patient signals consent by action, not verbally or in writing. From a nursing perspective, this may occur on a daily basis; a good examples is when a patient extends their arm forward for a vaccination or having their blood pressure and pulse measured. To avoid any misunderstanding, the nurse must always inform the patient what they require them to do and gain clarity as to what the person is actually consenting to. This advice may appear obvious, but it is very easy for a routine 'task' aspect of these procedures to override the nurse's duty to inform the patient of what procedure is being carried out. By contrast, expressed consent usually involves the patient signing a consent form, which provides a safe (but not conclusive) evidence that legal consent has been obtained. However, where such a form is not signed or has been amended without the patient's authorization, this leaves the medical practitioner open to a claim of non-consent to the procedure. Furthermore, if a patient has expressly consented to a procedure, and in the course of that procedure something else was done that was not immediately required, then the written consent to the original procedure may be no defence in a claim for trespass with respect to the additional procedure. Therefore, as affirmed in *Chatterton*, when a patient is asked to sign a consent form, it is necessary that they be given the chance to read and have explained to them what the consent form permits and does not permit, and be allowed to ask relevant questions concerning the proposed treatment. This should include sufficient warning of any potential risks of the medical/surgical procedure. The case of *Chester* (detailed earlier in Chapter 5) is an example of the key issues considered for a legal claim to be successful. It should be noted that a patient is free to withdraw their consent at any time; it would be unlawful for a medical practitioner or nurse to continue treatment unless it can be proved that the patient lacked capacity at the time of withdrawal.

For consent to be valid, the Department of Health (2009) stipulates that:

- It must be given voluntarily by: an 'appropriately informed person' who has the capacity to consent to an intervention; the parent or someone with parental responsibility for a patient under the age of 18; someone authorised with a Lasting Power of Attorney (LPA); or a Court Appointed Deputy with an authority to make treatment decisions.

- It must be given voluntarily and by a person under no duress, pressure or undue influence exerted upon them to either accept or refuse treatment.

- The person needs to understand the nature and purpose of the procedure, and any misrepresentation of such will invalidate consent.

In informed consent (also referred to as the prudent patient test), which originates from *Sidaway v Bethlem Royal Hospital Governors*, 'material risks' are determined and the medical practitioner discloses all such risks, giving the patient the opportunity to knowledgably evaluate the available options. Material risks are those that the medical practitioner knows are significant to the patient in making a decision as to whether to undergo the proposed treatment. In *Sidaway*, the Court also raised the matter of 'therapeutic privilege', an exception whereby the medical practitioner, following reasonable assessment, withholds information from the patient in cases where such disclosure may pose 'a serious threat of psychological detriment to the patient'.

In April 2007, the Act became legislation and has since provided a framework for supporting the autonomy of adults who either lack or have reduced capacity to make decisions. It holds that there be a statutory presumption that all adults have the capacity to make decisions, unless it can be shown that they lack the capacity to make a decision for themselves at the time the decision needs to be made (MCA, 2007). Prior to the Act and the Adults with Incapacity (Scotland) Act 2000, common law principles already existed to address matters of competence in decision-making. The Act has since served to establish such principles and embed them within statutory authority.

When trying to accept that a 'competent' patient wants to exercise their right to refuse treatment, in the first instance, it is important to note that competence is the ability to understand information about proposed treatment, such as its purpose, nature, likely effects, chances of success, potential risks and whether alternative treatments are available. Even if a patient considers the information differently from the health professionals, unwise choices are nevertheless permitted, as understanding does not necessarily imply a decision is made rationally. Many decisions are made by people on a daily basis via intuition or what is commonly termed 'gut-feeling'. The Act gives statutory recognition to unwise decisions in that they are not conclusive of a lack of mental capacity, but nevertheless reinforce the right to self-determination. Thus, like other healthcare professionals, the nurse may, in good faith, try to convince a patient otherwise; however, legally, they cannot, for example, compel the competent patient to eat, drink or accept other nursing or clinical interventions. The cases of *Re T, Re C* and *Re MB* addressed the issues of refusal and set precedent for later cases (Case studies 8.2).

Other notable cases that influenced common law concerning patient consent include *Chester v Afshar*, concerning the duty to warn patients about risk prior to obtaining consent (see Chapter 5); *Re B (Adult, refusal of medical treatment)*, the right of a patient with capacity to refuse life-prolonging treatment; and *St George's Healthcare NHS Trust v S, R v Collins and others, ex parte S* affirming the rights of a competent pregnant woman to refuse treatment even if such a refusal could result in harm to her or the unborn child.

CASE STUDY 8.2

RE T (AN ADULT: REFUSAL OF MEDICAL TREATMENT) [1992] 4 ALL ER 649

T was 20 years old and 34 weeks pregnant when she was involved in a road traffic collision and needed life-saving blood transfusion following a caesarean operation. Her mother was a Jehovah's Witness and had convinced her to observe her faith and sign a form refusing blood transfusions. Following the stillbirth of her baby, her condition deteriorated and she required ventilation. The doctor, her father and co-habiting partner (the child's father) applied to the Court to permit the medical staff to perform the transfusion. The Court subsequently ruled that the transfusion could be given, as the evidence had shown that at the time T decided not to have the transfusion, she did not have the required capacity to make a valid decision. Her altered competence led to a best interests decision to give blood to save her life and the baby's life.

RE C (AN ADULT: REFUSAL OF MEDICAL TREATMENT) [1994] 1 ALL ER 819

C was a patient with paranoid schizophrenia at a high-security hospital. He developed gangrene in his foot and his doctors felt that amputation was warranted. However, C refused to have the operation. Accepting that he had a condition which would probably result in his death if left untreated, he preferred to die as a complete man, believing that God would help him through his illness. The doctors argued that C suffered from delusions (including the belief that he was an international surgeon) and that therefore, he was unable to make a competent decision. C won his court case because the Court

Continued on following page

| CASE STUDY 8.2 | (Continued) |

believed he had mental capacity, as he was able to understand and retain information relevant to his treatment, and in believing the information, was able to arrive at a clear conclusion, irrespective of whether the decision was deemed good or bad.

RE MB (ADULT: REFUSAL OF MEDICAL TREATMENT) [1997] 2 FLR 426

MB required a caesarean section, but in a state of panic, withdrew consent at the last moment because of her phobia of hypodermic needles. The hospital was granted a judicial declaration that it would be lawful to carry out the procedure. Although MB appealed this decision, she later agreed to induction of anaesthesia and her baby was born by caesarean section. The Court of Appeal upheld the judge's opinion, that at the time, MB was not competent to refuse treatment, and due to her phobia, failed to weigh the information objectively. It viewed that her fear and panic had impaired her capacity to understand information she was given about her medical condition and the treatment advised. The judge reaffirmed the test of capacity set out in the *Re C* judgement. A person's capacity to make particular decisions may fluctuate or be temporarily affected by factors such as pain, fear, perplexity or the effects of pain-killing drugs. Thus, the assessment of capacity must be time and decision-specific.

Mental Capacity Act: Statutory Principles

Section 42 of the Act establishes the purpose of the Code of Practice, which provides guidance for those working within the legal framework of the Act and for those whose rights need to be addressed. This helps ensure that any decisions or actions taken are in the best interests of a person who lacks capacity to make a decision or act for themselves. The Act applies to those aged 16 and over, with Section 2(2) stating that the impairment or disturbance affecting capacity does not have to be permanent. Therefore, at the time a decision needs to be made, the loss of capacity can be partial or temporary, and the capacity can fluctuate over time. Additionally, a person may lack capacity to make a decision about one matter but not about others. The five statutory principles of the Act are the underpinning values that enable the fulfilment of the Act's ethos of being enabling and supportive, not restrictive and controlling. These are listed in Box 8.1.

As with other professionals, the nurse should use the following two-stage test (MCA Code of Practice, 2007) for assessing a person's capacity to make decisions for themselves:

1. Does the person have an impairment or disturbance of the mind or a brain that affects the way their mind works? Examples include dementia; significant learning difficulties; chronic brain damage; post-trauma concussion; some types of mental illness (e.g. psychosis); symptoms of alcohol/drug abuse; and medical conditions which may alter the level of consciousness.

2. Does the impairment or disturbance imply that the person is unable to make a specific decision when they need to? The Code of Practice (2007) describes that 'a person is unable to make a decision if they cannot':

   a. Understand the relevant information about the decision to be made. 'Every effort must be made to provide information in a way that is most appropriate to help the person to understand'. Relevant information includes the nature of the decision, the reason the decision is necessary and the likely effects of deciding either way or not making a decision at all. The capacity

BOX 8.1 ■ Five Statutory Principles of the Mental Capacity Act 2005

1. A person must be assumed to have capacity unless it is established that they lack capacity.
2. A person is not to be treated as unable to make a decision unless all practicable steps to help him/her to do so have been taken without success.
3. A person is not to be treated as unable to make a decision merely because he/she makes an unwise decision.
4. An act done, or made, under this Act on behalf of a person who lacks capacity must be done, or made, in his/her best interests.
5. Before the act is done, or the decision is made, regard must be had to whether the purpose for which it is needed can be as effectively achieved in a way that is less restrictive of the person's rights and freedom of action.

Adapted from the Mental Capacity Act, 2005. Code of Practice. Department for Constitutional Affairs 2007. TSO London.

for understanding is illustrated in *Re T* and expanded upon by the Court, stating that 'The more serious the decision, the greater capacity required'. The nurse needs to be mindful of the MCA, stressing the importance of giving information using the most effective form of communication. In consideration of the patient, using simple jargon-free language, sign language or pictures/diagrams and perhaps computer technology can help achieve better communication and enable effective decision-making.

b. Retain such information. 'The person must be able to hold the information in their mind long enough to use it to make an effective decision'. The use of notebooks, posters, photographs, videos and voice recorders may help people retain information. It must not be assumed that a person with a short memory span lacks the capacity to decide.

c. Weighing or using information to make the decision. At times, people can understand information but an impairment or disturbance may stop them from using it or lead them to make a specific decision without understanding or using the information they have been given.

d. Inability to communicate a decision. Such persons would include those who are unconscious or in a coma, and if there is no way a person can communicate their decision, the Act says they should be treated as if they are unable to make that decision. However, it is important to make all 'practical and appropriate efforts' to assist such persons to communicate. The nurse may need the assistance of other professionals, such as speech and language therapists or interpreters, to breach potential communication barriers. Other interventions may need to be considered; for example, a person with hearing difficulties may be familiar with visual aids, written messages or sign language, or a person with autistic spectrum disorder may communicate more effectively with the assistance of non-verbal assistive computer technology.

Capacity assessments are mostly related to one specific decision, but enduring conditions can affect people in making such decisions, particularly if that decision affects other decisions in their life. People may also have capacity that fluctuates, and renders it temporary due to their condition becoming worse on an infrequent basis. Bi-polar disorder is an illustrative example, as are other states, such as grief following a bereavement, post-traumatic shock or acute physical pain, all of which can adversely affect a person's decision-making capacity. For the nurse dealing with a patient suffering an enduring condition or a state rendering their capacity temporary, it is essential to consider the Code of Practice's emphasis on capacity being reviewed whenever a care plan is reviewed and developed, and when particular decisions need to be made. Any risk assessment must include the patient's understanding of risk and their ability/inability to weigh the information concerning particular decisions.

The 'Best Interests' Principle

Once it has been established that a person lacks capacity, the subsequent treatment and care must be in their best interests and refer specifically to the MCA Section 1, which states, 'An act done, or decision made, for or on behalf of a person who lacks capacity must be done or made in his (her) best interests'. Here, it is worth noting Kaplan et al.'s (2017) observation that the Act deliberately does not define 'capacity' by not specifying what is in a person's best interests, commenting that, '…it is a process that recognises that a conclusion that a person lacks decision-making is not an "off-switch" for their rights and freedoms… perhaps best be considered as a process of constructing a decision on behalf of the person who cannot make the decision themselves' (Kaplan et al., 2017). Their commentary emphasises the 2013 Supreme Court decision *of Aintree University NHS Hospitals Trust v James*, where it was stated that, 'The purpose of the best interests decision is to consider matters from the patient's point of view' and that 'decision-makers must look at his (patient's) welfare in the wider sense, not just medical, but social and psychological…'. This judgement dismissed the earlier Court of Appeal decision on the fundamental premise that it had, 'reached the right decision for the wrong reasons'. Sections 15–16 of the Act provide for the Courts to have powers to do for a person what they could do for themselves if they were of full capacity. For the reader, the judgement in *Aintree University NHS Hospitals Foundation Trust* merits further study, as it provides a useful point of reference for the underlying premise of 'best interests' decision-making.

Section 4 of the Act has an extensive 'best interests checklist', outlining what needs to be considered before making decisions or acting for a person who lacks capacity. The checklist must be referred to for any decisions, that avoid assumptions made on a person's age, appearance, condition or behaviour. A more concise adaptation of the best interests checklist is detailed in Box 8.2. Therefore, under Section 4, in assessing capacity and before deciding on a best interests decision, the assessor must consider:

- Whether it is likely that the person will regain capacity to handle the issue in question and when that is likely to be.
- As far as reasonably practicable, attempt to encourage the patient's participation or to improve their ability to participate in the process of decision-making.

> ## BOX 8.2 ■ Checklist: Best Interests Decisions on Behalf of Those Lacking Decision-Making Capacity
>
> 1. *Equal consideration* and *non-discrimination* of a person's best interests with no assumptions based on age, appearance, condition or behavioural characteristics.
> 2. *All relevant circumstances* relating to the decision in question concerning the person lacking capacity.
> 3. If the person is *likely to regain capacity*, for example, after receiving medical treatment, can the decision wait until after their recovery?
> 4. *Permit and encourage participation* as fully as possible from the person under consideration with regards to any act or decision that may affect them.
> 5. The *person's wishes and feelings* from past and present need to be considered, including those expressed verbally, in writing or through their behaviour or habits. Any religious, cultural, moral or political beliefs and values which may influence the decision should be ascertained.
> 6. Factors that include *the impact of the decision upon others* that the person would likely to consider if able to do so.
> 7. The *views of other significant people* regarding the person's best interests, such as a carer, close relative or friends who take a concern in the person's welfare. This may include any previously named person as someone to be consulted on the decision in question and associated matters. Any Lasting or Enduring Power of Attorney made by the person or a Court-of-Protection-appointed deputy to make decisions would need to be involved.
> 8. In cases concerning *life-sustaining treatment,* assumptions should not be made about a person's quality of life and neither should the decision be motivated by any desire to bring about the person's death.
>
> Adapted from Ruck Keene et al. (2020).

Exceptions to the principle of best interests are where a legitimate advance decision 'specific to the situation' has been made beforehand. Such a decision prevails even if it appears to not be in the patient's best interest. Additionally, under Sections 9–14 of the Act, where a Lasting Power of Attorney (LPA) is appointed with specific instructions given to them (as the donee) by the patient (as the donor) prior to the loss of capacity. The appointed donee has the power to make decisions for a person, both in terms of personal welfare (including consent or refusal to medical treatment) and of decisions relating to property and financial matters. It is possible to have more than one LPA, for example, one for financial and the other for healthcare decisions, and the donor can specify whether they should act independently or together. Should a situation arise in which two donees disagree, then arbitration is brought into being by the Court of Protection (COP). The COP was established with the jurisdiction to make decisions relating to a person's welfare, property and finance, and can make decisions with or without a court hearing; it can also appoint deputies with powers to make specific decisions on behalf of those over the age of 16 who lack the required mental capacity. Where a donor has created both an advance decision and an LPA, with specific instructions for the donee to be able to consent to or withhold specified treatments, then the advance decision will cease to be effective, because it would be considered that the donor no longer saw the advance decision as effective, as the LPA was drawn up after the advance decision.

Advance Directives

Regarding when a person lacks the requisite capacity, Maclean (2006) expanded upon the ideal of self-determination, affirming, 'If being in control of one's life is important, this loss of decisional-competence, whether temporary or permanent, will raise concerns as to how best to retain that control despite the envisaged period of incompetence. The desire to retain this control may be amplified by the current state of medical science, which is often capable of prolonging our survival in severely damaged and compromised states'. Thus, the attempt to control what happens to a person during an episode of incapacity is arbitrated through what is called an advance decision, also known as an advance directive, and, in lay-terms, known as a 'living will'. Brazier and Cave (2016) describe an advance directive as that which 'enables a person to set out his own instructions about any future treatment which he should, or should not, receive, were he to lose mental capacity to make such decisions for himself'. The MCA furthers that an 'advance decision' is a general principle of law and medical practice that people have a right to consent to or refuse treatment. It is detailed in Sections 24–26 of the Act. An advanced directive enables a person aged 18 or over to voluntarily refuse specified medical treatments. It may sometimes be viewed as a person preparing for old age, as with a will, or perhaps after a person has been informed that they have a specific disease or a life-changing medical condition. Healthcare professionals must follow advance directives and ensure that it is applicable to the patient's situation in question within current circumstances that fulfil the following criteria:

- That the proposed treatment is that specified in the advance directive.
- The circumstances are the same as those set out in the advance directive.
- That there are no changes in the patient's current circumstances which would have affected the decision made at the time they made the advance directive.

Generally, an advance decision is made in writing to provide documentary evidence, and although there is no set template, the Act advises that key information be provided. Such information would not only include the person's full name, signature, date of birth, home address and general practitioner (GP) details, but also a clear statement of the treatment decision to be refused and the circumstances in which such a decision applies. Furthermore, the advanced directive needs to be countersigned by a witness.

The nurse, as a healthcare professional, has the responsibility to be aware that a patient they intend to care for may have given an advance refusal to treatment, and that such valid and applicable advance decisions have the same legal status as those made by persons with capacity at the time of treatment. When discussing treatment options with the patient with capacity, the nurse should ask if there are any treatments they do not wish to receive, should they lack the capacity to give consent in the future. Additionally, speaking with the patient's relatives, looking in the hospital medical notes or contacting the patient's GP can assist the nurse in finding the existence of an advance directive for a patient who lacks capacity. The nurse must also be aware if an advance decision has not been reviewed or updated for some time, and if the patient's circumstances are notably different from those when the decision was made. If the healthcare team is unsatisfied regarding the validity and applicability of an advance decision, under Section 26 of the Act, they can still treat the patient under the 'best interests' principle, and should document why they did not follow the advanced decision. In such instances, the COP can resolve any disagreements about the validity and applicability of the advance decision when healthcare professionals have doubts over continuing treatment.

It is worth noting that a healthcare professional is protected from liability if they are unaware of the existence of an advance decision, or of failing to provide treatment if they reasonably believe that a valid and applicable advance decision to refuse that treatment exists. To demonstrate this belief, it has to be based on reasonable grounds and must be shown that the decision was made on evidence available at the time the decision was being considered.

Independent Mental Capacity Advocate (IMCA)

Established under the Act through new regulations in 2006, an Independent Mental Capacity Advocate (IMCA, 2006) is 'someone who provides support and representation for a person who lacks capacity to make specific decisions, where the person has no-one else to support them' (MCA, 2005). The IMCA makes submissions regarding the person's wishes, feelings and beliefs as factors to be brought to the decision-maker's attention. Detailed under Section 10 of the MCA Code of Practice, IMCAs provide service established under Section 35 of the Act. They are different from a normal advocacy service providers in that they serve those who have no one else to support or represent them, or where it would be inappropriate to consult others (for example, where there are concerns of abuse or coercion by family members or friends). An exception to this is when there are professionals or paid workers providing care and treatment, or if the person has not previously named someone who could assist with a decision or someone who has not been made an LPA. An IMCA is a trained person appointed by the Local Authority (in England) or Health Board (in Wales), and can assist with information gathering for the patient and their relatives and/or carers for the benefit of best interest assessment, as well as with identifying others who should be contacted. An IMCA can assist families steer through the process of best interest assessment, and ensure that the patient's views and wishes are actively heard.

Situations where an IMCA must be instructed include the following:

- Where an NHS body is proposing to provide, withhold or stop treatment that is likely to have serious consequences for the patient or when the choice of treatments is finely balanced between benefit and risk.

- Where an NHS body or Local Authority is proposing to arrange or change accommodation for the patient in a hospital for 28 days or more.
- Where an NHS body or Local Authority is proposing to arrange accommodation in a care home for the patient for more than 8 weeks.

Exceptions to these instructions would be when an urgent decision of a life-saving nature has to be made; for example, chemotherapy and surgery for cancer; major limb amputations; withholding artificial nutrition and hydration; and Electro-Convulsive Therapy.

Neither the Act nor its Code of Practice specifies precise time periods to review capacity or best interests decisions. However, reviews should take place either when developing the patient's care plan or when the patient's condition changes materially and key decisions need to be made (British Medical Association, 2019). Therefore, the nurse needs to ensure that detailed records of all reviews and changes to the patient's treatment and care are made and stored safely.

Medical Paternalism and the Influence of *Montgomery*

Paternalism can be defined as 'the policy of governing... in a paternal way... fatherly... limiting freedom by well-meant regulations' (Concise Oxford Dictionary, 2011). Although a number of models of nursing exist with a non-medical and philosophical foundation that link theory to practice, in many respects, nursing still follows the pathway and practices driven by doctors known as the medical model. In the ethical debate concerning medical paternalism, Robinson and Doody (2021) emphasise an approach that makes a distinction between three different forms of paternalism: *Hard* – direct coercion, for example, law; *Soft* – which entails giving unasked for information or foreclosing some options for actions; and *Maternalism* – which involves psychological control, for example, targeting a sense of guilt. An example of *hard* paternalism could be that all children up to 135 cm tall or between the age of 3 and 12 must wear an appropriate child restraint if travelling in the front seat of a car. An example of *soft* paternalism and *maternalism* could be that of a healthcare professional advising that casual sex between two persons should involve the use of physical protection, such as a condom, to prevent the possibility of contracting a sexually transmitted disease. Thus, whilst not removing choice, this enables making a healthier choice centred on responsibility.

Medical paternalism reflects a position that is opposite to accepting a patient's right to autonomy, even though its object is 'good' and has the same moral status as independence. It implies that the medical practitioner makes decisions on what they determine are in the patient's best interests, even for those patients who are able to make their own decisions. In recent years, this 'doctor knows best' attitude has come under harsh criticism in aspects of the doctor-patient relationship. Although it could be argued that paternalism really means beneficence, Brazier and Cave (2016) purport that a professional judgment on what is good for the patient requires that the medical practitioner 'still ultimately… accepts her (his) decisions on what is good for her (him).'

The Supreme Court decision concerning the case of *Montgomery* (discussed earlier in Chapter 5) challenged this historical paternalism and set precedent for later decisions influencing case law throughout the UK. The decision is summarised in Case 8.3 as follows.

Key factors in the Supreme Court decision of *Montgomery* are summarised as follows:

CASE STUDY 8.3	**Montgomery v Lanarkshire Health Board [2015] UKSC 11**

Brief summary: Mrs Montgomery (M) had her baby delivered vaginally, but it was born with cerebral palsy as a result of occlusion of the umbilical cord caused by a form of obstructed labour, shoulder dystocia. She sued the NHS Trust, claiming that the Consultant Obstetrician knew she was a diabetic and that the baby would have been larger than average; consequently, she should have informed her of the risk of this condition developing, and have given her the option of a caesarean section, which would have circumvented these risks and prevented the child's permanent injury.

The judgement: The lower court (Court of First Instance in Scotland) supported the General Medical Council and rejected Mrs Montgomery's argument in applying the Bolam test; this decision was also upheld by the Inner House of the Court of Session (Scotland). M appealed to the Supreme Court, which, after reviewing the law on informed consent, upheld her appeal in that a breach of duty of care had existed.

- A revisiting of the decision in *Sidaway*, in that a particular approach was seen as too pivotal upon the doctor and one that could absolve a doctor of liability if they had followed a small body of practice that could support the decision made. Therefore, an emphasis upon what a patient 'would want to know' is advised and that the doctor not only provides information (e.g. clinical risks), but facilitates the understanding of such information given (Turton, 2019).
- It is a patient's fundamental right to make their own decisions relating to their medical treatment, and that there has been a shift towards personal autonomy since *Sidaway*, whereby *Sidaway* was viewed as not reflecting reality. Society was now 'pointed away from a model of the relationship between the doctor and the patient based upon medical paternalism'.
- If a patient suffers injury as a result of an undisclosed risk that a doctor showing reasonable care would have disclosed, then the injured patient would have a claim in negligence.
- Patients undergoing procedures which would have a 'profound effect' on them should be advised of alternative treatments.
- The Human Rights Act and European Court of Human Rights (ECtHR) has moved away from medical paternalism and further recognised a person's right to self-determination.

Heywood (2015) provided critical commentary on the questions raised about *Sidaways'* continuing validity and appropriateness, and of the House of Lords' reliance for many years on the case as the leading authority on disclosure; that it was allowed to continue for so many years before being overruled by the Supreme

Court in *Montgomery*. As described by Chan et al. (2017), *Montgomery* was seen as 'a clash of values – patient autonomy versus medical paternalism'. From an ethical viewpoint, *Montgomery* clarified the prevailing shift towards a more cooperative approach between doctors and patients, where patient autonomy is now more valued in treatment decisions. Even though the ruling in *Montgomery* did not radically change the process of consent, it has nevertheless been described as having 'simply given appropriate recognition to patients as decision-makers' (Chan et al., 2017).

References

Brazier, M, Cave, E, 2016. Medicine, patients and the law, 6th ed. Manchester University Press, Manchester.

British Medical Association, 2019. Best interests decision-making for adults who lack capacity: A toolkit for doctors working in England and Wales. Available at: https://www.bma.org.uk/media/1850/bma-best-interests-toolkit-2019.pdf.

Chan, SW, Tulloch, E, Cooper, ES, Smith, A, Wojcik, W, Norman, JE, 2017. Montgomery and informed consent: where are we now? British Medical Journal 12 (357) J2224.

Department of Health, 2009. Reference guide to consent for examination or treatment. Available at, 2nd ed. https://www.gov.uk/governement/publications/reference-guide-to-consent-for-examination-or-treatment-second-edition.

Herring, J, 2018. Medical law and ethics, 8th ed. Oxford University Press, Oxford.

Independent Mental Capacity Advocates, 2006. The Mental Capacity Act 2005 (General Regulations 2006). Available at: https://www.legislation.gov.uk/uksi/2006/1832/pdfs/uksi_20061832_en.pdf.

Kaplan, M, Doyle, S, Campbell, P, 2017. A brief guide to carrying out best interests assessments. Essex Chambers. Available at. https://www.39essex.com.

Maclean, AR, 2006. Advance directives, future selves and decision making. Medical Law Review 14 (3), 291–320.

Mental Capacity Act (MCA) 2005. Code of Practice. Department for Constitutional Affairs 2007. TSO London.

Nursing and Midwifery Council, 2018. The Code: professional standards of practice and behaviour for nurses, midwives and nursing associates.

Robinson, S, Doody, O, 2021. Nursing & healthcare ethics, 6th ed. Elsevier, Oxford.

Ruck Keene, A, Butler-Cole, V, Allen, N, Lee, A, Kohn, N, Scott, K, Barnes, K, Edwards, S, David, S, 2020. Determining and recording best interests. 39 Essex Chambers. Available at. https://www.39essex.com/mental-capacity-guidance-note-best-interests-july-2020/.

Taylor, H, 2018. Informed consent 1: legal basis and implications for practice. Nursing Times 114 (6), 25–28.

Turton, G, 2019. Informed consent to medical treatment post-montgomery: causation and coincidence. Medical Law Review, 27(1), 108, pp 1–25.

Oxford Dictionaries, 2011. Concise Oxford dictionary, 12th ed. Oxford University Press, Oxford.

Oxford Dictionaries, 2018. Oxford dictionary of law, 9th ed. Oxford University Press, Oxford.

CASES

Aintree University NHS Hospitals Foundation Trust (Respondent) v James (Apellant) [2013] UKSC 67
Chatterton v Gerson [1981] 1 All ER 257
Chester v Afshar [2004] UKHL 41
Montgomery v Lanarkshire Health Board [2015] UKSC 11
R (Burke) v GMC [2005] 3 FCR 169
Re B (Adult, refusal of medical treatment) [2002] 2 All ER 449
Re C (An Adult: Refusal of Medical Treatment [1994] 1 All ER 819
Re T (An adult: refusal of medical treatment) [1992] 4 All ER 649
Re W (a minor: medical treatment) [1992] 4 All ER 627
Sidaway v Bethlem Royal Hospital Governors [1985] 1 ALL ER
St George's Healthcare NHS Trust v S, R v Collins and others, ex parte S [1998] 44 BMLR 160

STATUTE

Adults with Incapacity (Scotland) Act 2000
Mental Capacity Act 2005

The Law and Children's Welfare

KEY TERMS

Child protection

The Children Act 1989 and 2004

Safeguarding

Court orders

Children and Social Work Act 2017

Gillick competence

Introduction

The protection of children is a global priority, and the United Nations Convention on the Rights of the Child (UNCRC, 1989) and the Human Rights Act (1998) have raised the importance of countries complying with international law concerning the rights and welfare of children. In the UK, the Children Act 1989 provides a structure for the establishment of services for vulnerable children, laying down the principles to be followed when deciding upon the welfare of the child. Children who are neglected or abused have an increased likelihood of adverse long-term consequences, including mental health problems, reduced educational achievement, substance misuse and criminal behaviour. At 16 years of age, a child is presumed to be competent according to the law, thus enabling them to give consent to (or refuse) their treatment. However, at the age of 16–17, a child who lacks the capacity to consent may be treated without their consent under the Mental Capacity Act, so long as a deprivation of liberty is not implicated. Treatment can also take place within the bounds of the legal concept of 'parental responsibility', as laid down by the Children Act 1989.

Legal Aspects of Child Welfare

This chapter provides a brief overview of the law within England; Wales, Scotland and Northern Ireland have similar legislations concerning the welfare and protection of children. For the purposes of the Children Act 1989 and Family Law Act 1996, a child is regarded as a person under the age of 18. In observing that the Children Act 1989 places a general duty on local authorities to promote and safeguard the welfare of children in need in their jurisdiction, Foster (2020) reiterates that the Act sets out what a 'local authority must do when it has reasonable cause to suspect that a child in the area is suffering, or is likely to suffer harm'.

Under Section 3 (1) of the Children Act 1989, parental responsibility is defined as 'all the rights, powers, responsibilities and authority which by law a parent of a child has in relation to the child and his property'. This responsibility inevitably applies to the mother, unless she forfeits these rights or is proven incapable of applying such rights. The law pertains to the father if he is married to the mother at the time of insemination or birth; however, if he is not married to the mother, then under the Family Law Reform Act 1987, he can acquire parental responsibility either by marrying the mother or if the child's birth was registered after 1 December 2003. Additionally, under the Adoption and Children Act 2002, he can acquire such responsibility if he registers as the child's father on the birth certificate. An unmarried father may be appointed as the child's guardian following the mother's death and acquire parental responsibility; to confirm such rights, documentary evidence is required, such as a court ordered parental responsibility agreement or a marriage certificate. In case of parents' divorce, the parental responsibility remains under Section 2 of the Children Act 1989; Section 4 of the Children Act 1989 has the provision that enables step-parents to take on parental responsibility if all parties reach an agreement. However, such an agreement does not remove responsibility from those for whom it already exists. Parental responsibility is only terminated if the child is given up for adoption. Nevertheless, such responsibilities can fall short as regards providing a safe, nurturing environment for children to thrive in and remain healthy. Consequently, a legal framework is necessary for those with parental responsibility as well as those in authority within the health and social care system. The Children Act 1989 was formed to reflect the UNCRC 1989, in that the welfare of children was paramount, with local councils having a duty to carry out enquiries (often urgent) under Section 47 of the Act, where there was 'a reasonable cause to suspect that a child who lives in their area is suffering, or is likely to suffer significant harm'.

The implementation of the Children Act 1989 in providing an effective legal framework for the safety and protection of children incorporates the following five central principles.

1. The <u>welfare principle</u>, which is determined by a court considering the following checklist as laid out in Section 1 of the Children Act:
   a. The ascertainable wishes and feelings of the child to be considered in relationship to their age and understanding to make a wise choice on the matters concerned (See *Gillick v West Norfolk and Wisbech AHA* later in the

chapter). If the child lacks maturity and understanding, then the court may appoint a guardian or an independent officer of the Children and Family Court Advisory Service to act in the interests of the child.

b. The child's physical, emotional and educational needs that go beyond their social class, affluence or perceived happiness.

c. The likely effect caused upon a child by a change in circumstances. For example, one parent leaving the family home.

d. The age, gender and background of the child can be influential and would include the basic feeding, housing, clothing and physical and psychological care as well as the child's educational interests and being able to make decisions for themselves.

e. Any harm the child has suffered or is at risk of suffering.

f. The capability of the parents and others to meet the child's needs.

2. The principle of <u>keeping the family together</u> is based on the presumption that a child is best looked after within a family where both parents play an equal part. Rather than take an oppositional stance with families experiencing adversity, social services departments are advised to support the role and duties of the family rather than consider removing the child in the first instance. According to this principle, the Children Act 1989 (Section 17) defines a *child in need* as one that is 'unlikely to achieve or maintain a reasonable standard of health or development without the provision of services by a local authority or their health development is likely to be significantly impaired or further impaired without the provision of services by a local authority or they are disabled'.

3. The <u>non-intervention</u> principle presumes that the court should not intervene, that is, make an order unless it is in the best interests of the child and serves to maintain the self-determination and veracity of the family. An example is a divorce case in which the parents agree that the child live with one parent but spend alternate weekends with the other parent.

4. The need to <u>avoid delays,</u> where a child is at risk and where applications for court orders need to be applied for and timetabled towards a resolution of a case. Additionally, when prolonged legal processes may prejudice the welfare of the child in question.

5. The <u>unifying of laws and procedures</u> was created by the Children Act 1989 to provide a single set of legislations which include legal resolution of disputes within families (private matters) and public law matters concerning protecting children from harm. This unification of law is concisely described in the Scarman lecture by the President of the Supreme Court, Lady Hale (2019). A three-tier court system was thus created in terms of the level of complexity and seriousness, from the Magistrates' Family Proceedings Court to the County Court and then to the High Court, where adoption cases and appeals from the Family Proceedings Court may need to be heard.

The catalysts for developments following the Children Act 1989 were the inquiries into the deaths of Victoria Climbié and Baby P (see Case studies 9.1 and 9.2),

CASE STUDIES 9.1 AND 9.2	Inquiries into the deaths of Victoria Climbié and Baby P

9.1 VICTORIA CLIMBIÉ

Victoria Climbié, an 8-year-old, died in February 2000 as a result of murder by her great-aunt and her aunt's boyfriend. Victoria had suffered months of abuse and neglect resulting from torture and starvation. Such brutal acts included cigarette burns, tying her up and repeated beatings with chains and belt buckles from which multiple injuries were evident. The inquiry, chaired by Lord Laming and the subsequent report – Laming Report (Laming, 2003) – revealed that up to Victoria's death, the NHS, police, NSPCC, local church and the social services departments across four local authorities were all in contact with her and had noticed signs of abuse. At the murder trial, the judge pronounced that 'blinding incompetence' had led to this failure by the services. The Laming Report condemned not only the failings of individual professionals, but also of senior organisational managers in being accountable for their departments and accepting responsibility for failing to take appropriate protective action for Victoria.

9.2 BABY P

Peter Connelly (Baby P) was 17 months old when he died in August 2007 as a result of months of abuse carried out at home by his mother, her live-in boyfriend and the boyfriend's brother. Baby P had suffered multiple injuries over an eight-month period, including breaks in his back, shinbone and ribs; his finger-tips being cut off; nails pulled out; and a tooth swallowed. Numerous agencies were involved with Baby P and his family. In December 2006, he was placed under child protection/at risk register, and over the following months, he had been admitted to hospitals and placed in temporary care as a safeguarding measure. Following Peter's death, the perpetrators were imprisoned; the subsequent case review reports highlighted serious failings by the local child protection services, including a lack of 'professional curiosity' and a reliance on the accounts of Baby P's mother; furthermore, there was a lack of transparency by medical professionals, as they did not attend his child protection meetings to provide insights into the severe nature of his injuries. Poor responses by professionals and lack of awareness by social services workers who were looking after Baby P, were viewed as significant failings.

as a result of which the Children Act 2004 and the Laming report offered significant recommendations. A further report by Lord Laming gave an analysis of problems facing local councils and resourcing challenges such as recruiting and retaining social workers (Laming, 2009).

Lord Laming's enquiry into the murder of Victoria Climbié and subsequent recommendations led to the founding of the Children Act 2004, which established a standardised approach to improve the way in which services work together to provide early help for families. Under Section 11 of the Act, responsibility was on the safeguarding partners to work together and be more accountable to promote the safety and welfare of children in their locality. Historically, state intervention in the lives of children had been focussed on the 'risk or reality of significant harm' being done to children. The important change signalled by the Children Act 2004 was the concept of promoting welfare of all children and introducing it into UK law (Green, 2019). Coinciding with the 2004 Act was the government publication, 'Every child matters: change for children', which specified national priorities for children's services. It outlined a framework of outcomes for children and young persons as well as greater ministerial responsibility overseeing the strategic implementation of these new priorities. To work within a regulatory framework, new directors within local authorities were created to oversee children's services, as were Local Safeguarding Children's Boards, or LSCBs (2006, 2010) (HM Government, 2006) throughout England and Wales. The scope of LSCBs had a wider remit than the previous child protection system; it aimed to identify and prevent maltreatment or impairment to the health and development of children and proactively work towards targeting particular groups of vulnerable children and responding to protect those children who are suffering or are at risk of harm. Overall, the LSCBs had a statutory duty to ensure the collective accountability of agencies and organisations working within the processes of child protection under Section 47 of the Children Act 1989. The LSCBs were replaced following the Children and Social Work Act 2017, which also amended the Children Act 2004; the new partnership comprised the police, health providers and local councils, working under the new *Working Together to Safeguard Children* guidance (2018).

Significant court cases concerning child protection include *Z and Others v The United Kingdom,* concerning a breach of Articles 3 and 13 of the ECtHR regarding the neglect of four children who had been living in filthy conditions, suffering 'appalling' neglect in their parent's home; *E and others v The United Kingdom*, concerning an infringement of Articles 3 and 13 of the ECtHR, where four children were abused by their stepfather, and there was negligence of the local services in failing to protect the children; *A and Another v Essex County Council,* where a local authority, during the adoption process, failed to inform the adoptive parents of the child's violent behaviour and serious psychological difficulties; *R v BS*, concerning a man beating his children and step-children and other physical abuse over a protracted period of time; and *R v Townsend-Oldfield*, where three girls between the ages of 12 and 14 were enticed by a woman into her home for the purpose of her common-law husband indecently assaulting and raping them.

THE CHILDREN AND SOCIAL WORK ACT (CSWA) 2017

The CSWA amended the Children Act 2004 with the following key changes:
- Safeguarding partners were the central component, with the local authority, clinical commissioning groups (CCGs) and police forces determining how safeguarding arrangements should work in their area for them and relevant agencies, both statutory (e.g. NHS and NSPCC – a charity with statutory functions) and non-statutory (e.g. Action for Children), who play a vital role in coordinating the safeguarding and welfare of children.
- Under Section 16 of the CSWA.

To regulate the relevant agencies that safeguarding partners may choose to work with and to establish the roles and responsibilities of the safeguarding partners:

- Requires that local safeguarding partners make arrangements to identify serious child safeguarding cases which raise issues of importance to the area, and where arrangements for the children are to be supervised.
- Requires that local safeguarding partners publish their arrangements and ensure independent scrutiny of how effective the arrangements are, thereby ensuring the duty of safeguarding partners to act in accordance with the published arrangements.
- Requires for people/bodies to supply information to the safeguarding partners, if requested, to enable or assist in their functions.
- To establish a Child Safeguarding Practice Review Panel to 'identify serious safeguarding cases which raise issues that are complex or of national importance and to arrange, where appropriate, for those cases to be reviewed under their supervision'. Such reviews aim to identify improvements required to safeguard and promote the welfare of children.
- Local Authorities have a duty to notify the panel if a child: has either been abused or neglected; dies or is seriously harmed in the locality; or dies or is seriously harmed outside England while normally resident in the Local Authority's area.

Child Protection and Nurse's Duty

Vulnerability (derived from Latin *vulnerabilis)* implies that there is a greater risk of an adverse event concerning people's health, safety and well-being (Bailie and Black 2015). Vulnerable children and young people face an increased risk of being subjected to abuse and/or neglect and 'by its very nature, child abuse is often hidden from view and many cases don't come to the attention of the police or the courts' (Office of National Statistics, 2020). Wilkinson and Bowyer (2017) add that there was an increased risk of child and adolescent maltreatment when parents contended with their own vulnerability. Examples of such factors include a history of crime; acrimonious separation between parents; domestic abuse; mental health difficulties and/or substance misuse.

As with other health and social care professionals, the nurse too has a moral, ethical and professional duty to report any potential harm or abuse that they suspect is happening with those they come in contact with, as well as with those patients that provide direct care for. Although no single piece of legislation in England concerns the promotion and safeguarding of children's welfare, there exists a multitude of regulations and laws. However, in certain occupations that involve work with children, such as nursing, there is an expectation that a professional has an obligation to fulfil the principles encompassing a 'duty of care', which includes a duty to report known or suspected abuse and neglect. At a professional level, the NMC 'Code' (2018) is clear about the nurse's responsibility to 'take all reasonable steps to protect people who are vulnerable, or at risk from harm, neglect or abuse' (Part 17, NMC

Code, 2018). This protection requires the nurse to share information regarding a person deemed at risk in line with the laws concerning disclosure of information, as well as possessing the knowledge and observing the relevant laws and policies about protecting and caring for vulnerable persons.

If a nurse is worried that their employer or another organisation is not responding to or sharing child protection information appropriately, it is essential that the concerns be aired for the benefit of the child's safety. In certain cases, the nurse may be led to 'whistle-blow' if it is reasoned to be in public interest; this can help prevent an organisation from operating without regard for the safety of others, including children. Whistle-blowing can also promote transparency and compliance. In England, Scotland and Wales, it is protected by law under the Public Interest Disclosure Act 1998, which was inserted into the provisions of the Employment Rights Act 1996. The *Working Together to Safeguard Children* statutory guidance reflects the NMC's Code stating that 'anyone who has concerns about a child's welfare should make a referral to local authority children's social care and should do so immediately…' (HM Government, 2018). Although this guidance does not impose an absolute legal requirement to comply, it requires the nurse to take it into account; if they depart from it, the nurse must have clear reasons for doing so.

Within the NHS, the frontline of leadership concerning child safeguarding is provided by designated and named professionals. Indeed, it is a requirement for each provider to have an established named doctor and nurse and for clinical staff to have access to such persons. The designated professional's duties are '…to provide advice to health organisations regarding planning, strategy, commissioning and performance indicators with regard to safeguarding service provision and to help with appropriate audit of practice guidance and policies….' (Green, 2019). Clinically, these designated professionals can provide advice on the legal aspects of child protection, in addition to documenting and critically evaluating evidence, writing reports and presenting information in child protection meetings. The designated nurse usually works at a senior consultant level, having completed specific training with considerable experience in the care of babies, children and young people and an understanding of forensic medicine. In complex cases, they may also have to resolve matters of dispute between professional workers. The different types of child abuse are summarised in Table 9.1.

Child Protection – The Duty of the Courts

If a child is suspected of suffering significant harm, or likely to suffer harm, the Children Act 1989 provides for legally-binding protection arrangements through applications to the Courts (see Box 9.1).

Medical Treatment: Consent in Children

For the purposes of consenting to medical treatment, under the Family Law Reform Act 1969, English law has a special rule for those who are aged 16 or over (but not yet 18), who, with their consent, can be administered medical treatment in opposition

TABLE 9.1 ■ Types of child abuse

Physical
May involve hitting, shaking, throwing, poisoning, burning or scalding, drowning or suffocating to cause harm. Such harm may also be caused when a parent/carer fabricates the symptoms of or deliberately induces illness in a child.

Emotional
That which has a persistent, adverse effect on the child's emotional development and may involve the child feeling unloved, worthless, inadequate and not able to express their views. The child may be deliberately silenced or have fun made of when they do communicate. This may also involve age or developmentally inappropriate expectations being imposed and interactions beyond a child's developmental capability, as well as overprotection and the child being limited in how they explore, learn and participate in normal social interaction. Bullying (including cyber-bullying) would be included here, as well as the child witnessing the ill-treatment of others and/or frequently feeling frightened and in danger.

Sexual
Involves forcing a child or young person to take part in sexual activities, which may include assault by penetration (e.g. rape or oral sex) or acts such as kissing, masturbation, rubbing and touching outside of clothing. Non-contact activities are also included, such as looking at or being involved in producing sexual imagery and watching sexual activity, including online imagery. These acts can be committed by women as well as other children. Sexual exploitation of the child is where the child is groomed through being given gifts, including money and affection, in exchange for taking part in sexual activities. Such activities can involve violent, humiliating assaults by multiple perpetrators. The child may be tricked into believing they are in a loving, caring relationship with their abuser and not fully aware of the nature of the abuse.

Neglect
This is a persistent failure to meet a child's physical and psychological needs, likely to result in the serious impairment of the child's health and development. It can include substance abuse during pregnancy as well as a child not being provided with adequate food, clothing and shelter or being abandoned. Neglect also includes parents' or caregivers' failure to protect a child from harm or danger and providing inadequate care and supervision, including failure to ensure access to medical care and treatment.

Child Trafficking
(Modern Slavery)
Involves recruiting and moving children either within or from outside the UK for the purposes of either sex exploitation, benefit fraud, forced marriage, forced labour, domestic servitude or forced crime, such as transporting drugs or pickpocketing. Children who are trafficked often experience all the forms of abuse listed above and become part of organised criminal networks. A child cannot legally consent to their exploitation, so only the evidence of movement is required and not that of the abuse that they have endured. Child trafficking is dealt with under the auspices of the Modern Slavery Act 2015.

Female Genital Mutilation (FGM)
FGM is a criminal offence and involves the removal of external female genitalia (by circumcision) for non-medical reasons. It is carried out within infancy as well as childhood, adolescence and just before a woman is married or during her pregnancy.

Adapted from Working Together for Children 2018 and NSPCC Learning 2020.

BOX 9.1 ■ Children Act 1989 – Child Protection Arrangements

Public law. Under Section 17 of the Child Protection Act 1989 (hereon the 'Act'), a duty is placed on local authorities (hereon referred to as LAs) to provide in their area a range of appropriate services to promote and safeguard the welfare of children in need; due consideration should also be given to the child's wishes. A *child in need* is defined as one who (a) Is unlikely to achieve or maintain, or to have the opportunity of achieving or maintaining a reasonable standard of health or development without the provision of LA services; (b) will have their development significantly impaired, or further impaired without the provision of LA services; (c) is disabled. Section 20 of the Act places a duty upon a LA to provide accommodation (voluntary arrangement) to a child in need if they require it due to either no one having parental responsibilities of the child; or the child is lost or abandoned; the person caring for them is prevented from providing reasonable accommodation or care; the child has reached the age of 16 and their welfare is likely to be 'seriously prejudiced' if they are not provided with accommodation. Such a child is termed a 'looked-after child'.

Section 47 of the Act establishes what LAs must do to protect children at risk of harm, and in the first instance the LA must make the necessary enquiries to decide whether it should act to safeguard or promote a child's welfare. Other bodies, such as the Clinical Commissioning Group or Local Housing Authority also have a duty to assist the LA in conducting such enquiries. Situations which require these enquiries would be when the LA has been informed that a child in their area is the subject of an Emergency Protection Order or is in police protection. Enquiries are also made if the LA has 'reasonable cause to suspect that a child who lives, or is found in their area is suffering, or is likely to suffer significant harm'.

Under Section 31 of the Act, a 'looked-after' child on the application from the LA or NSPCC (as an authorised person) may be subject to the court making a supervision or care order. However, the court needs to be satisfied that the child concerned is suffering, or likely to suffer significant harm and that the harm is attributable to the child being beyond parental control and/or the care that the child is receiving is not what being it would be reasonable to expect a parent to give them. A care order places a child in the care of the LA and a supervision order places a child under the supervision of an LA where the LA must 'advise, assist and befriend' the child, but not having parental responsibility. Section 1(3) of the Act provides a 'welfare checklist' for assisting with decision-making when effecting care/supervision orders, and this checklist also pays regard to the wishes of the child as well as their identified needs.

Emergency protection orders are provided for under Section 44 of the Act, such an order may be made following application by any person, and that the court is satisfied that there is good reason to believe that a child is likely to suffer significant harm if they are not removed to different accommodation provided by or on behalf of the applicant, or that the child does not remain in the place in which they are being accommodated. Under Section 47 of the Act, this type of order can be made by a LA application if the court is satisfied that enquiries are being obstructed and access to the child is being unreasonably refused, and where that access is urgently needed. This is a temporary order which lasts for 8 days but it can be extended on one occasion for a further 7 days.

Continued on following page

BOX 9.1 ■ Children Act 1989 – Child Protection Arrangements (Continued)

Private Law – Section 8 Orders.

Under Section 8 of the Act, there are three orders which can be made in any family court or care proceedings:

- *Child Arrangement Order* where it is decided that arrangements for whom a child is to live with, spend time with or otherwise have contact with and when a child can spend time or have contact with any person. If an agreement can be reached regarding the arrangements for whom a child is to reside with or spend time, then a consent order can be applied for. This informal agreement is legally binding and enforceable through the Family Court.
- *Prohibited Steps Order* which is granted by the court to prevent one parent from exercising their parental responsibility in a way that is not in the child's best interests.
- *Specific Issues Order* which gives directions for the purpose of deciding upon a specific question which has arisen, or which may arise in connection with any aspect of parental responsibility for a child. Examples could be that of whether the child should have religious education, certain medical treatment or when the child should attend school.

Adapted from Foster, D., 2020. An overview of child protection legislation in England. House of Commons Library Briefing Paper No. 6787).

---

to their parents or guardian's consent; the medical practitioner will not incur any liability under civil or criminal law. However, the Family Law Reform Act does not apply to cases concerning organ donation or procedures which are non-therapeutic or are for the purposes of research. The Mental Capacity Act confirms that those young persons between the age of 16 and 18 will be treated as adults for the purposes of the Act, with the exception of those who are unable to make an LPA or an advance decision. Described as a 'landmark case', *Gillick v Norfolk and Wisbech AHA*

CASE STUDY 9.3	**Gillick v West Norfolk and Wisbech Area Health Authority [1986] AC 112 HL**

In Gillick v West Norfolk and Wisbech AHA, Victoria Gillick, a mother of five daughters, challenged a DHSS circular which advised that in certain circumstances, contraceptive advice and prescribing could be sought and given to persons under the age of 16 without parental consent. She took court action, arguing that it was unlawful and contrary to a doctor's legal obligation in that the child was below the legal age at which she could lawfully consent to intercourse, and adversely interfered with parental rights and duties in terms of actions against their knowledge and wishes for the child. The Department of Health (2003) refused to give her assurances that none of her children would be given contraception without her permission. Mrs Gillick failed in the High Court, but won in the Court of Appeal, only to have the judgement reversed by the House of Lords, where although Lord Fraser acknowledged that the parents should normally be asked, he nevertheless stated:

'Provided the patient, whether a boy or a girl, is capable of understanding what is proposed, and of expressing his or her own wishes, I see no good reason for holding that he or she lacks the capacity to express them validly and effectively and to authorise the medical man to make the examination or give the treatment which he advises. After all, a minor under the age of 16 can, within certain limits, enter into a contract. He or she can also sue and be sued, and can give evidence on oath. I am not disposed to hold now, for the first time, that a girl aged less than 16 lacks the power to give valid consent to contraceptive advice or treatment, merely on account of her age...'

is a prime example where perceived parental rights and responsibilities conflict with a child who has the capacity to exercise their autonomous right to consent to medical advice and treatment. See Case study 9.3 (below).

Gillick was later re-affirmed in *R (on the application of Axon)* where the court also stated that parental consent was not necessary for contraception, treatment of sexually transmitted disease or abortion if such treatment was in the child's best interests and they had consented to such interventions. The implication that the doctor had aided or abetted a girl in having unlawful sexual intercourse was concretised in the Sexual Offences Act 2003, where a medical practitioner serves to protect a child from becoming pregnant or contracting a sexually transmitted disease, and also to protect the child's physical safety and emotional well-being. Although *Gillick* was not a unanimous decision by the House of Lords, it did affirm that a minor was capable of consenting to treatment if they demonstrated 'sufficient understanding and intelligence' about what was being proposed. This factor of a child's maturity provides the point of decision-making in what has since been referred to as 'Gillick competence' within medical and family law. In accordance with the decision made, Lord Fraser laid down more detailed criteria for a doctor to consider when assessing a child's competence, which are interpreted as follows:

That the doctor…

- is satisfied that the child understood the advice.
- is prepared to attempt to persuade the child to tell their parents or let the doctor do so. Only if the child refuses would the doctor then be entitled to continue with the treatment.
- is of the opinion that the child was very likely to have sexual intercourse with or without contraceptive advice or treatment.
- is of the opinion, that unless the child got the advice, their physical or mental health would suffer.
- is sure that the child's best interests required the advice without the knowledge or consent of the parents.

The matter of a child under the age of 16 having the maturity to understand and appreciate the consequences (short- and long-term risks and benefits) of consenting to a particular medical procedure were put to the test in the case of *Re R (A Minor: Wardship; Medical Treatment)*. In Re R, a child was detained under the Mental Health Act 1983 and had refused to take antipsychotic medication; the child had a mental illness, which was intermittent in nature, resulting in intermittent *Gillick* competence upon which the child's decision relied. Therefore, as the Court of Appeal would not apply *Gillick* to a patient with fluctuating capacity, treatment was ordered in accordance with the best interest's obligations under the Children Act 1989. Although *Gillick* evolved from the background of contraceptive counselling, it submitted that the court's ruling on the capacity of a child under 16 was applicable to other forms of medical intervention as well. However, '*Gillick mature*' to 'consent' does not necessarily apply to *Gillick mature* 'to refuse to be treated' as such a refusal can be overridden by the parents/guardians or the court on the grounds that either they have a coexisting legal capacity to consent; that such a refusal might possibly lead to serious harm or death; and that the child may not be able to fully understand the consequences of their refusal.

Gillick: Ethical Considerations

Gillick raises considerable debate around the ethical pillars of autonomy, confidentiality and beneficence. The daughter had a right to self-determination and make an autonomous decision as a competent child, along with the right to a confidential discussion (including treatment advice) with the medical practitioner. Her best interests were deemed to be integral to the decision made by her medical practitioner on the grounds of necessity. The medical practitioner must calculate the balance between respecting a young person's confidentiality to maintain trust and the importance of protecting that young person from harm. But what if that course of breaching confidentiality aggravates the risk of harm? A deontological perspective would judge the morality of that breach of confidence by whether the action in itself was right or wrong, based on a broader system of rules, including that of the medical practitioner doing their duty and abiding by the principles of the Hippocratic Oath. By contrast, a consequentialist perspective would argue that the morality of respecting confidentiality is based exclusively on all the good that it fosters as well as the harm that arises if it is breached, calculating a harm/benefit ratio of consequences. Preserving confidentiality may benefit the young person by encouraging disclosure of all relevant clinical information, thereby enabling the clinician to act more effectively while being mindful that when a substantial risk is identified, then breaching confidentiality and sharing information with parents and other professionals may reduce the risk of harm.

The principles of beneficence were presented in *Gillick* and the 'for' and 'against' views well-described by Brazier and Cave (2016), summarised as follows:

- *For.* That if significant numbers of young girls under sixteen are going to have sexual intercourse, regardless of whether they have legal access to contraception, it may be in their best interests to protect them from pregnancy by contraceptive treatment.
- *Against.* As purported by Victoria Gillick, if access to contraception without parental agreement was prevented, at least the majority of young girls would be deterred from starting to have intercourse so young for fear of pregnancy and/or parental disapproval. This may also serve as a defence from peer pressure to engage in sexual intercourse as part of 'growing-up'.

Common ground for agreement was that under-age contraception helps prevent diseases, such as venereal disease or cervical cancer, as well as any potential for future mental health damage that the child may undergo.

The right to confidentiality lies in the young person's right to autonomy and the freedom to make meaningful choices about their own health. The deontological perspective lies with the choice not being ultimately 'good' or 'bad', but in the innate freedom to make that choice. It could be argued that developing autonomy and individuality helps young people transition towards adulthood by taking responsibility for their own health and welfare. It also assists parent or guardians to view this increasing independence as part of their child's emotional and psychological development. Respecting these ethical principles also serves to remind the nurse to be mindful of their own ethical values and cultural background, highlighting that subjectivity will always play a part in how a nurse may judge the autonomy of children as patients, just as they would do with adult patients.

The Incompetent Child Under the Age of 16

In the case of a patient who is under the age of 16 but not *Gillick competent*, legal consent to the medical treatment rests with the patient's parents or guardians. Parental responsibility is defined under Section 3(1) of the Children Act 1989 as, 'all the rights, duties, powers, responsibilities and authority of which by law a parent of a child has in relation to the child and his property'. Consent needs to be only given by one parent/guardian; however, it is legally advisable and good clinical practice for the medical practitioner to involve both parents. Such parental rights are extensive but not absolute, and in particular circumstances, they do have limitations. For example, changing a child's name or school requires the agreement of each parent, and if this cannot be made, then the court determines the matter. Therefore, parental responsibility exists for the child's benefit; the concept of child's best interests, today, has a broader meaning than just medical matters. The case of *Re R (a minor) (Blood transfusion)* illustrates the court's powers to exercise its judgement in the best interests of the child. This case concerned the refusal of the parents, both of whom were devout Jehovah's Witnesses, for their 10-year-old daughter to receive a blood transfusion. The local authority sought an order under Section 8 of the Children Act 1989 for the transfusion to be given; taking into consideration the parents' religious beliefs, the Court nevertheless ruled for the child to receive the treatment, as her situation was life-threatening. A latter case of *NHS Trust v Child B and Mr and Mrs B* involving the child of Jehovah's Witness parents, who had suffered severe burns, delivered the same judgement, on the grounds of the child's best interests. This state interference to protect a child's welfare is made under the old doctrine of *parens patriae* (Latin, 'father of the people') where, in English Law, the family courts are given the authority of parents, to represent the interests of those children that require protection. However, in the more complex case of *Re T (a minor) (Wardship: Medical Treatment,)* a different judgement was made following a reversal by the Appeal Court. A two-year-old child (T) was moved abroad by his parents, whom he lived with. The parents had concluded that he should not be subject to the liver transplant that was advised for his life-threatening medical condition. The local authority intervened and sought a court order for T's return to the UK for the transplant; however, the parents asserted that even if the transplant was successful, the child would be subject to further pain and distress and would have to take anti-rejection drugs for the rest of his life, possibly facing further surgery. The Court of Appeal allowed the mother's refusal to stand in favour of the child having a short happy life, being cared for by his mother with the financial and emotional support of his father and a peaceful death. This was preferred to him enduring a considerably unhappy life, where he would be taken into care with continued medical intervention.

The Case of *Re A (Minors) (Conjoined Twins: Separation)*

As outlined in Chapter 4, this unique case concerned Jodie and Mary (pseudonym of the conjoined twins), where a number of ethical and legal issues were deliberated. Such issues arose from a tragic moral dilemma, which attracted global media attention and considerable debate amongst the public and academics as well as the legal and medical professionals. The beliefs and religious convictions of the twin's parents were considered to merit great respect, but the court could not avoid the responsibility of deciding the matter to the best of its judgement regarding the twins' best interests.

Both twins had the intrinsic right to life and rights to bodily integrity and autonomy. In this case, autonomy meant the right to have one's own body, whole and intact, and on being of an age to understand and be able to take decisions about the same. The court did not value J's life above M's; however, M's death would be because her body could not survive on its own. Therefore, M's death was viewed as an inevitable consequence of an operation that was necessary to save J's life. Furthermore, continued life for M would mean pain and discomfort for however long she lived. The proposed invasive surgery was seen as a positive act. Nevertheless, academic commentary raised such central questions as, 'When does a human being become a person and worthy of respect as such?'; 'What role can the characteristic of physical separation play in establishing such status?'; 'When, if ever, should considerations of "quality of life" be allowed to outweigh those of "sanctity of life" ?'; 'Who should decide what is in the best interests of a child, for example - parents, doctors or the courts?'; and 'What factors should be taken into account in making this decision?' (Sheldon, 2001). The doctrine of double effect was a key concept in the separation of the twins, which is defined by Pearn (2001) as '...the fact that some actions have unavoidable bad effects as well as good...that actions might be ethically justified if: the bad effects were thought unfortunate and regrettable, the bad effects would not outweigh the good effects, the action were not intrinsically bad, i.e. independent of its effects and the bad effects were not the means of the achievement of the good effects'. Emphasising that the twins' parents were competent and not negligent, Gillon (2004) expressed that the court should have 'declined to deprive the parents of their normal responsibilities and rights in order to impose its own preferred resolution of the moral dilemma and should have allowed the parents to refuse medical intervention – while still ruling that such separation should not have been unlawful had the parents consented'.

In contrast to the decision in *Re A (minors) (conjoined twins: separation)*, a more recent case of baby Charlie Gard generated considerable global interest and reflected discordant views embedded in different philosophies of parental authority, life and medical care. Once again, there was considerable debate among medical practitioners, religious leaders, academics and the general public. Charlie Gard's case is outlined in Case study 9.4.

CASE STUDY 9.4	**Great Ormond Street Hospital for Children NHS Foundation Trust v Yates and Others [2017] EWCA Civ 410**

Charlie Gard (C) was an 11-month-old baby who died in a hospice in 2017 having suffered a rare genetic condition called mitochondrial DNA depletion syndrome (MDDS), where he could not move his limbs or breathe on his own. His parents, Chris Gard and Connie Yates, wanted C to be transferred to the USA to undergo an experimental treatment, as there were no treatments available in the UK for MDDS. The Great Ormond Street Hospital in London said that treating C's disease would be futile in that it would prolong his suffering; this was endorsed through a second opinion by an expert medical team from Spain. The court upheld the hospital's decision on 'best interest' grounds and C's transfer to the USA was refused. The parents appealed through both the Court of Appeal and Supreme Court, but this too was unsuccessful. Eventually, the U.S. specialist medical practitioner, following further MRI scans of C, declined to offer further help. C's parents then relinquished their efforts to transfer C, despite believing that it might have helped, had their child been transferred sooner.

At this stage, C's parents wanted to take C home to die, or to a hospice; however, the hospital initially refused this on the basis that C's medical needs were too complex and that a hospice could not provide the kind of intensive life support necessary to keep C alive for a few more days. Soon after, however, the hospital doctors agreed for C to be transferred to a hospice with removal from life support.

Gard – Ethical and Legal Debate

The *Gard* case prompted a call for legal reform of substituting the *best interests* test with a *significant harm* test, believing this would strengthen parental rights and ensure that mediation was offered in the more contentious cases. This proposal was known as 'Charlie's Law'. A similar case around the same time was that of *Alder Hey Children's NHS Foundation Trust v Evans and others*, concerning baby Alfie Evans, which prompted similar legal reform known as 'Alfie's Law'. Both these cases involved a conflict between the wishes of parents to preserve their children's lives and the judgements of their medical teams in pursuit of clinically appropriate therapy. In both cases, the treatment required was extraordinary and entailed the provision of a wide array of advanced life-sustaining technological support. The proposed reform had three elements: (i) a focus on assisting parents to gain better access to ethical advice and their rights; (ii) for parents to get independent second opinions and legal aid, particularly if taking on high-level legal representation; and (iii) the protection of parental rights in these cases by preventing court orders being made, with the exception where there is a risk of significant harm to the child. The courts must suppose that responsible, caring parents make reasonable and satisfactory decisions for the good of their children, instead of focusing on hypothetical best interest's judgements made by the courts. Nevertheless, it must be considered that if parents act unreasonably or malevolently, their wishes could be overridden; the medical professionals have the right to conscientiously object towards carrying out procedures that may be regarded as unnecessary or harmful.

However, this reform did have opposition. Positing why the proposal to substitute the *best interests* test with *significant harm* test should not happen, Benbow (2020) offered four considerations: (i) such a reform would make UK law inconsistent with international law, in that creating a harm threshold would be incompatible with the ECtHR, which requires the child's best interests to be the paramount consideration of welfare institutions and the courts; (ii) parents are not always the best people to make decisions regarding their children's medical treatment because their emotional state of grief or hopes for their child may make them disposed to not accept the limitations of the medical and surgical treatment available; (iii) the proposal could adversely impact the distributive justice approach, where limited medical resources are being consumed on experimental treatment for a child, when the same level of financial funding could be allocated to a greater number of children who would benefit from proven effective treatments. This underpins the rule utilitarian ethical principle of striving to create the greatest good for the greatest number of people; and (iv) if parents cannot find doctors to treat their children in accordance with their wishes, this would be unworkable, as many cases have confirmed that the courts will not compel a doctor to treat as there is no legal requirement, despite the parent's own beliefs and motivations.

Parental Control

The concept of the zone of parental control (ZPC) was introduced in 2008, and is provided for in the Mental Health Act 1983: Code of Practice (Department of Health, 2015) concerning patients under the age of 18. However, as Taylor (2018) notes regarding this definition, 'the Code does not limit its application to treatment for mental disorder. Practitioners would therefore be well advised to apply it generally to all treatments'. Concepts concerned with its application include who has parental responsibility, and what it means for children/young persons to be capable of consent. The rights, powers and duties associated with parental responsibility apply until a child/young person attains *Gillick* competence. Once it is ascertained who has parental responsibility, the person responsible for the patient's care and treatment must determine whether that person has capacity under the MCA to take decisions about a child/young person's treatment and whether that decision falls within the ZPC. Therefore, in assessing whether a particular decision sits within the limits of the ZPC, lawyers and clinicians should be mindful of the two key questions identified by the Code of Practice:

1. An objective question – Is this a decision that a parent should reasonably be expected to make? Factors to consider would include:
   - Whether the child/young person lacks Gillick competence.
   - The type and invasiveness of the proposed intervention. The more extreme the intervention, the more likely it will lie outside the ZPC, and greater justification would be needed for treating the child/young person.
   - The age, maturity and understanding of that particular child/young person.
   - The extent to which the child/young person agrees or resists.
   - Any relevant human rights decisions of the courts.

2. A subjective question – Are there any indications that the parent might not be acting in the best interest of the child/young person, which might undermine the validity of this person's consent? Factors to consider would include:

- A parent who is incapacitated.
- A parent who is unable to focus on the best interests of the child/young person.
- A parent who is overwhelmingly distressed by the situation or other external factors that may affect their decision-making ability.
- Those parents who are not in agreement.

Ultimately, the court can give consent to any treatment decision provided it is in the child's/young persons' best interests, and it resolves any disputes as to whether treatment is in the child's/young person's best interests. The nurse must be aware that the law concerning consent to medical treatment develops continually with the increasing maturity and advancing autonomy of children/young persons. Even though the law in England and Wales generally reveres and upholds the European Convention and UNCRC, disputes occasionally arise between a child's/young person's acknowledged rights to self-determination, and that of the paternalistic welfare concerns of parents and the courts.

References

Baillie, L, Black, S, 2015. *Professional values in nursing*. CRC Press, London.

Benbow, DI, 2020. An analysis of Charlie's Law and Alfie's Law. Medical Law Review 28 (2), 223–246.

Citizens Advice, 2021. Court orders to protect children. Available at: https://www.citizensadvice.org.uk/family/children-and-young-people/protecting-children/court-orders-to-protect-children/.

Department of Health, 2003. Every child matters: green paper. Available at: http://www.educationengland.org.uk.

Department of Health, 2015. Mental Health Act 1983: Code of Practice. Available at: https://assets.publishing.service.gov.uk/government/uploads/system/uploads/attachment_data/file/435512/MHA_Code_of_Practice.PDF.

Foster D, 2020. An overview of child protection legislation in England. House of Commons Library Briefing Paper No. 6787.

Gillon, R, 2004. Jodie and Mary, conjoined twins: a case of judicial moral hubris? Medico-Legal Journal 72 (Pt.1), 3–16.

Green, P, 2019. Symposium: child abuse. The role of designated and named professionals in child safeguarding. Paediatric and Child Health 29 (1), 1–5.

Hale L, 2019. 30 years of the Children Act 1989. Scarman Lecture 13/11/19, Law Commission. London. Available at: https://www.supremecourt.uk/docs/speech-19113.pdf.

HM Government, 2006. Working together to safeguard children: a guide to interagency working to safeguard and promote the welfare of children. The Stationery Office, London.

HM Government, 2018. Working together to safeguard children: a guide to interagency working to safeguard and promote the welfare of children (updated July 2018). The Stationery Office, London.

Laming, L, 2003. The Victoria Climbie Enquiry: report of an enquiry by Lord Laming. Norwich. The Stationery Office. CM 5730.

Laming, L, 2009. The protection of children in England: a progress report. The Stationery Office, London. HC330.

Local Safeguarding Children's Boards Regulations, 2006. SI 2006/90.

Local Safeguarding Children's Boards Regulations, 2010. SI 2010/622.

Nursing and Midwifery Council, 2018. The Code: professional standards of practice and behaviour for nurses, midwives and nursing associates.

Office of National Statistics, 2020. Child abuse and the Criminal Justice System, England and Wales, year ending March 2019: Information on response to and outcomes of child abuse cases and the criminal justice system. Available at: https://www.org.gov.uk.

Pearn, J, 2001. Bioethical issues in caring for conjoined twins and their parents. The Lancet 357 (9272), 1968–1971.

Sheldon, S, 2001. On the sharpest horns of a dilemma': re A (conjoined twins). Medical Law Review 9 (3), 201–207.

Taylor H, 2018. Children – which decision counts? Available at: https://bevanbrittan.com/insights/articles/2018/children-which-decision-counts/.

United Nations, 1989. United Nations convention on the rights of the child. Available at: https://www.unicef.org.uk/.

Wilkinson J, Bowyer S, 2017. Research in practice: the impact of abuse and neglect on children; and comparison of different placement options: evidence review, March 2017. Department for Education Reference: DFE – RR663.

CASES

- A and Another v Essex County Council [2003] EWCA Civ 1848
- Alder Hey Children's NHS Foundation Trust v Evans and others [2018] EWHC 953 (Fam)
- Airedale NHS Trust v Bland [1993] AC 789
- E and others v The United Kingdom [2002] ECtHR 33218/96
- Gillick v West Norfolk and Wisbech Area Health Authority [1986] AC 112 HL
- Great Ormond Street Hospital for Children NHS Foundation Trust v Yates and Others [2017] EWCA Civ 410
- NHS Trust v Child B and Mr and Mrs B [2014] EWHC 3486 (Fam)
- R v BS [2010] EWCA Crim 2691
- R (A Minor; Wardship: Medical Treatment) [1992] 3 Med. L.R. 342
- R (on the application of Axon) v Secretary of State for Health [2006] EWHC 37 (Admin)
- R v Townsend-Oldfield [2010] EWCA Crim 2451
- Re A (Minors) (conjoined twins: separation) [2000] Lloyds Rep. Med.425.
- Re A (Conjoined twins) [2001] 2 WLR 480
- Re R (A Minor) (Blood transfusion) [1993] 2 FLR 757
- Re T (a minor) (Wardship: Medical Treatment) [1997] 1 All ER 906
- Z and Others v The United Kingdom [2001] 2 FLR 612

STATUTE

- Adoption and Children Act 2002
- Children Act 1989
- Children Act 2004
- Children and Social Work Act 2017
- Family Law Reform Act 1969
- Family Law Act 1996
- Family Law Reform Act 1987
- Human Rights Act (1998)
- Sexual Offences Act 2003

End of Life Care – Legal Aspects

KEY TERMS

Death

Sanctity of life

Euthanasia

Withdrawing treatment

Assisted suicide

DNR orders

Introduction

It is essential for nurses to understand what end-of-life care entails, as part of the individual care-planning process, and that the involvement of the patient with decision-making is fundamental to such care. The NMC Code (2018) Standard 3.2 states that it is a duty of the nurse to 'recognize and respond compassionately to the needs of those who are in the last few days and hours of life'. Nurses caring for patients at the end of life often face ethical and legal challenges that may make them feel uneasy or distressed, particularly if they view their work as that of principally preserving life. There is no legal obligation to either start or discontinue life-sustaining treatment if it is no longer in the patient's best interests to do so; indeed, it is unlawful to either start or continue treatment against a person's wishes. For those patients who lack capacity, the Mental Capacity Act (MCA) sets out specific mechanisms, amidst the ethical predicament of the principle of the *sanctity of life* versus the patient's *quality of life*. The quandary faced by medical professionals has resulted in court interventions. This chapter gives a brief overview of notable cases. With increasing longevity of human life, nurses are faced with caring for an increased number of ageing persons within the domestic population in both hospital and community settings. They must remember that even though English law does not essentially distinguish between younger and older adults, the Human Rights Act 1998 still applies. This chapter focuses on the law specifically concerning adults.

Death – The Medical Perspective

The General Medical Council (GMC) describes persons approaching the 'end of life' as those who are likely to die within 12 months, including:

- those whose death is imminent within a few hours or days
- those with advanced, progressive, incurable conditions
- general frailty and co-existing conditions where death is expected within 12 months
- existing conditions if the person is at risk of dying from a sudden acute crisis in their condition
- life-threatening acute conditions caused by sudden catastrophic events
- extremely premature neonates whose survival prospects are deemed to be very poor
- patients diagnosed as being in a persistent vegetative state (PVS) for whom a decision to withdraw treatment may lead to their death.

Taken from GMC (2020) Treatment and Care towards the end of life: good practice in decision making

Although there is no statutory definition of death, the Academy of Medical and Royal Colleges (AMRC, 2008) state, 'Death entails the irreversible loss of those essential characteristics which are necessary to the existence of a living human person and, thus, the definition of death should be regarded as the irreversible loss of the capacity for consciousness, combined with the irreversible loss of the capacity to breathe'. This irreversible cessation of the brainstem function – 'brainstem death' – has become the gauge for deciding whether a person is dead. Brainstem death follows cessation of cardiorespiratory function (cardiac arrest) and the absence, for a period of time, of blood circulation to the brain. Testing for the absence of brainstem and cough reflexes, as well as motor responses are the essential aspects required for a diagnosis of brainstem death. For a decision to cease attempts to resuscitate a patient, the AMRC outlines criteria primarily predicated upon whether previous attempts of applying cardiopulmonary resuscitation have failed and/or 'treatment aimed at sustaining life has been withdrawn because it has been decided to be of no further benefit to the patient and not in his/her best interest to continue and/or is in respect of the patient's wishes via an advance decision to refuse treatment' (AMRC, 2008).

However, regarding a patient in an irreversible state whose breathing is artificially maintained by a ventilator machine, the decision in the case of *Re A*, concerning a ventilated child, provides an interesting illustration as to whether the medical practitioner who had disconnected the ventilator had acted unlawfully. Most decisions concerning the treatment of a person at the 'end of life' are dealt with by medical professionals; however, the nurse too has specific duties to the dying person. The nurse's duties would benefit from being aligned to the priorities of care, listed based on work by the Leadership Alliance for the Care of Dying People (2014), which followed an independent review with Neuberger (2013) who highlighted the importance of recognising the needs of a dying person. The review emphasized that communication and decisions should be made in accordance with the dying person's needs and wishes, and that care must regularly be reviewed and revised within an individualised care plan that is delivered compassionately. Other priorities include communicating sensitively with the dying person and those important to them, in addition to involving such persons in the treatment and care decisions. Nurses caring for patients at the end of life are often confronted with uncomfortable ethical and legal issues, such as deciding to discontinue life-sustaining treatment, for instance, clinically assisted nutrition and hydration (CANH); they may also be reluctant to administer an opioid for pain relief because they fear it might act as a respiratory depression and speed up the patient's death.

Sanctity of Life

The concept of *sanctity of life* is a religious moral conviction about how human beings are to be perceived and treated – an ideological, virtual-ethics concept. Much has been studied and written by philosophers and theologists, but Baranzke (2012) concisely describes the religious foundation of sanctity of life as being that 'life is a gift from God' and the non-religious view that life merits 'the upmost respect with which human life should be treated'. In exploring this concept, Baranzke (2012) refers to the earlier work of Frankena (1975), who made the distinction between an *absolute* respect for life – meaning that all life-shortening acts are morally wrong, and *qualified* respect for life – where some life-shortening acts are permissible. Baranzke (2012) also considered the writings of Kuhse (1987), who gave a non-religious definition from the absolute perspective that, 'it is absolutely prohibited either intentionally to kill a person or intentionally to let a patient die, and to base decisions relating to the prolongation or shortening of human life on considerations of its quality or kind'. Historically, the law throughout the United Kingdom has been obligated to these Christian principles; however, some court cases have recognised situations where the non-natural continuation of the life of a patient does not always serve to enhance that patient's life. Indeed, Heywood and Mullock (2016) argues that this traditional concept of *sanctity of life* so closely aligned with religious beliefs now suffers from the weakness that 'religion no longer dictates the contours of the criminal law'. Brazier and Cave (2016), in emphasizing that the medical profession acts within the constraints of criminal law of murder and manslaughter, state that issues of life and death are left to such common law due to a 'political disinclination to engage in debate on the sanctity of life'. World-renowned philosopher Ronald Dworkin held that 'most people who are not religious also have general, instinctive convictions about whether, why, and how any human life has intrinsic value' (Dworkin, 1994), which constitute a secular (non-spiritual) deep philosophical belief. However, the concept of *sanctity of life* has its supporters and opponents. Herring (2020) makes the distinction in 'that life in, and of itself is valuable. Even if a person is in a coma, with no awareness of the outside world and with no friends or relatives to be concerned about them, has value by virtue of being human'. Opposing this view is the belief that, 'what makes life valuable are the things that people do with it. It is the experience people have, their relationships and activities which give life meaning' (Herring, 2020).

Adult patients with capacity have the absolute right to decide whether to accept treatment. Where such a voluntary informed decision is made, it must be acknowledged by the nurse, even if it results in the patient's death. It is unlawful for the medical practitioner to give treatment in such an instance. However, 'basic or essential care' would be expected throughout a patient's illness, suffering and subsequent stay in hospital, as defined by the Mental Capacity Act Code of Practice (2007). The notion of *suffering* is very wide-ranging, and has 'not been traditionally regarded as a legal concept, but mainly as the psychological underpinning of human rights violations' (Andorno and Baffone, 2014). The case of *B v An NHS Trust* illustrates the autonomy of a patient (paralysed from the neck down) with decision-making capacity to have the legal right to request for their ventilator to be switched off. In this case, the medical practitioners refused, and subsequently, the patient brought a successful court action against the healthcare trust on the grounds of battery. Eventually, the patient was allowed to die. Where the adult patient lacks decision-making capacity, any decision to withdraw life-sustaining treatment must be shown to be in the patient's best interests. The case of *Aintree University Hospitals Foundation Trust v James* illustrates this context.

Withdrawal of CANH

In the first instance, it is important to understand the difference between an act and an omission. *Airedale NHS Trust v Bland* is a leading landmark case which provides an example of a working understanding of the difference between the two approaches (Case study 10.1).

In B's case, it could be argued that switching off the life support machine was an *act*, as was removing the naso-gastric feeding tube. However, the House of Lords disagreed with this, viewing it as an acceptable *omission*. They stated that '…essentially what is being done is to omit to feed or ventilate; the removal of the naso-gastric tube or the switching off of a ventilator are merely incidents of that omission'. Thus, CANH was viewed as part of medical treatment and not deemed 'basic care'. The decision in Bland could be viewed as a moral one that required careful justification in legal terms, given the possibility of being viewed as endorsing euthanasia. As Szawarski and Kakar (2012) pointed out, '…cultural and religious beliefs or legal restraints will continue to impact on withholding of assisted nutrition and hydration… it is likely to be defined by the anti-euthanasia lobby as a form of "killing" and by the remainder of society as pragmatic and potentially "inhumane"'. Whereas there was considerable debate before the House of Lords gave their decision, the view from Tony Bland's parents held, that if he was in a position to voice an opinion, he would not have wanted to live in his current state; this held despite an absence of evidence to support this declaration, as Tony had

| CASE STUDY 10.1 | **Airedale NHS Trust v Bland [1993] AC 789** |

At 17 years of age, Tony Bland (B) was left in a persistent vegetative state after sustaining crush injuries at the Hillsborough Stadium football match. He was kept alive for three years with a life support machine, but showed no signs of recovery. Technically, he was still alive, as his brain stem was still functioning, which controlled his heartbeat, breathing and digestion via a naso-gastric tube. He required full care, as he was not conscious. Following consent from his parents, the hospital applied for a declaration to lawfully discontinue life-support procedures to keep 'B' alive in that state, including withdrawing his artificial ventilation, nutrition and hydration. The House of Lords granted the declaration, recognising an intention to cause death and end B's suffering, even though euthanasia was not lawful. The decision was appealed by B's solicitor, but this was dismissed, as the doctor's duty was deemed to act in B's best interests on the basis that with no potential for improvement, maintaining treatment was futile. The court considered that the withdrawal was not an act but an omission of treatment; in B's circumstances, it was considered lawful to withdraw his nutrition and withhold life-prolonging treatment for a person who had no prospect of having any quality of life. Ten days after the withdrawal of his nutrition and hydration, B passed away.

not voiced any opinion on the subject before incurring his injuries. The law lords required that treatment have no therapeutic purpose for it to be regarded as futile, and that keeping the patient's best interests by continuation of life preserving treatment was rebuttable. Therefore, the sanctity of life principle was no longer a default position if it was considered that the patient's life no longer has any meaning, value or quality. Similar to other more recent cases, the Tony Bland case illustrates how much the courts are influenced by medical evidence and the clinical opinion of medical practitioners when making their judgements. Different considerations and legal judgements may be made concerning those patients who are in a clinically diagnosed minimally conscious state – where they show clear but minimal or inconsistent awareness, with periods where they can communicate or respond to commands by movement (e.g. a finger) when asked. The cases of *An NHS Trust v DJ and others* post-operative multi-organ failure) and *W v M and others* (mother of a brain-damaged woman) illustrate that the continuation of life-sustaining treatment for patients in a minimally conscious state may be judged as beneficial, leaving open the prospect of recovery.

Euthanasia and Assisted Suicide

Oxford Dictionary (2018) defines 'euthanasia' as 'The act of taking life to relieve pain. …voluntary… where the sufferer's life is ended at his or her specific request…and non-voluntary, where a person is unable to express his or her wishes…e.g. a person in a Persistent Vegetative State, and involuntary, where a person is killed without his own or any proxy authority'. Involuntary euthanasia is always illegal, whereas voluntary and non-voluntary euthanasia, regardless of compassionate motives, depend on whether the act is *active* or *passive*. Active euthanasia is illegal because steps are actively taken to assist in suicide (e.g. by administering a fatal drug), thus amounting to murder. By contrast, passive euthanasia is considered legal if carried out in the patient's best interests, as in the *Bland* case. Because euthanasia is not recognised by law in England and Wales, there is a distinction between killing a person and letting them die. Although no longer unlawful to take one's own life, under the Suicide Act 1961, Section 2(1) as amended by the Coroners and Justice Act 2009, it is unlawful for another person to assist or encourage a suicide; such an action may be liable for prosecution by the courts.

According to Herring (2020), encouraging suicide involves urging or supporting another person to take their own life (whether or not the person actually does). To be guilty of the offence, the defendant must intend to encourage another person to commit or attempt to commit suicide. Any defence for the act of 'mercy killing' cannot be relied on, as the law does not recognise such a defence. Additionally, Herring (2020) notes that the defence of diminished responsibility has been recognised in very few cases brought before the courts with resulting manslaughter convictions; indeed, a conviction for gross negligence manslaughter would arise if a healthcare professional or carer acted in an extremely negligent manner. Nevertheless, the implications of those persons who wish to assist a relative or friend to take their own life extends to the motivations of healthcare professionals who wish to end the painful suffering of a patient in their care. A patient may seek assistance from a nurse to help them end their life; however, the nurse must reflect on their own ethical and professional codes of practice, as well as the broader moral and legal obligations. For example, it would be unwise for a nurse to advise a patient to go abroad to end their life or if the patient is considering an overdose, inform them of what amounts to a fatal dose, as this would be considered assuming the right to assist another to commit suicide.

The primary aim of prohibiting assisted suicide is to protect vulnerable persons from being coerced into taking their own life by unprincipled relatives or friends. The plight of Dianne Pretty and the ensuing legal case received international attention, addressing the reasoning and judicial decisions of the 'right to die' under the canopy of the Human Rights Act (Case study of 10.2).

The later landmark case of *R (on the application of Purdy) v DPP* took a different direction from *Pretty* and was the last case to reach the appellate committee of the House of Lords (now the Supreme Court); although similar to *Pretty*, it led to a different outcome. See Case study 10.3.

As Chahal (2009) highlighted, *Purdy* overruled the decision in *Pretty* by engaging Article 8, thereby sparking a fresh debate regarding 'assisted suicide'. Indeed, 'public interest' was influenced via public morality, even though assisted suicide remains a criminal offence. Therefore, despite the DPP issuing a Code for Crown Prosecutors (DPP, 2010) on those travelling abroad for assisted dying as well as assisted dying in England and Wales, ultimately, the courts must decide on judgements and sanctions based on each individual case. Official figures from the Crown Prosecution Service (CPS) show that from 1 April 2009 to 31 July 2021, 171 cases, referred to the CPS by the police, have been recorded as assisted

CASE STUDY 10.2	**Pretty v United Kingdom [2002] 2 FLR 45**

Dianne Pretty (D) suffered from motor neurone disease which causes progressive muscle wasting, loss of normal body movement and serious difficulties with speech, swallowing and breathing. There is no cure and it leads to a slow death. D was at an advanced stage of the condition – she was paralysed from the neck down, hardly able to speak and required tube feeding. Fearing that she would suffer a slow and undignified death, she appealed to the Director of Public Prosecutions (DPP), seeking her husband's immunity from prosecution under Section 2(1) of the Suicide Act 1961, should her husband assist her to die. This was refused, which led D to seek judicial review of the decision in the High Court, along with the right to decide the time and circumstances of her death. The High Court found for the DPP, as did the House of Lords on appeal. D claimed that the DPP's refusal was a breach of the European Convention Articles 2 (right to life), 3 (freedom from inhuman and degrading treatment), 8 (right to respect for private life), 9 (freedom of conscience) and 14 (freedom from discrimination). On this premise, D then appealed to the European Court of Human Rights, but the court deemed that there was no violation; thus, the appeal was unsuccessful. Article 2 confers a right to protect (the sanctity of) life and does not give a right to die; Article 3 did not extend to ensuring that a terminally ill person, unable to take their own life, was entitled to seek the assistance of another person without being exposed to prosecution by law. Essentially, Article 3 includes a right to live with dignity, not die with dignity. Furthermore, Article 8 did not suggest that a person had the choice to no longer live, as it is directed at persons having their autonomy protected to live their life.

CASE STUDY 10.3	**R (on the application of Purdy) v DPP [2009] UKHL 45**

Debbie Purdy (P) suffered multiple sclerosis, due to which her physical state was degenerating to the point she feared she might wish to end her life, but would not be able to do so because of her physical disability. She decided she wanted assistance from her husband to end her life when the time came. Even assisting P to travel to a Swiss Clinic to gain lawful assistance to die would mean that her husband, or any helpers, would be liable to prosecution and imprisonment under Section 2 (1) of the Suicide Act 1961. For P, this was not an acceptable consequence, as she wanted a guarantee that her husband would be immune from prosecution. P made a High Court action against the DPP, charging that it had infringed on her human rights under Article 8 of the European Convention, which gives the right to respect for her private life and a qualified guarantee that there would be no interference by a public authority in exercising this right. P argued that there was a lack of specific guidance on assisted suicide in the Code for Crown Prosecutors; however, the High Court and the Court of Appeal did not rule in P's favour. Consequently, in 2010, the House of Lords backed P's argument, even though it did not rule as to whether assisted suicide was lawful. The House of Lords ordered the DPP to end the uncertainty by pronouncing new and more transparent policy guidance upon physician-assisted suicide, as well as that of a loved one assisting a sufferer to travel to a facility for this purpose.

suicide. Of these, the CPS did not proceed with 111, and 32 were withdrawn by the police (CPS, 2021).

The DPPs Code for Crown Prosecutors (2010) consists of a two-stage test – an evidential stage and public-interest stage, which comprises a list of factors favouring prosecution as well as factors against prosecution. Factors 'against' include:

- the victim had reached a voluntary, clear, settled and informed decision to commit suicide;
- the suspect was wholly motivated by compassion;
- the actions of the suspect, although sufficient to come within the definition of the offence, were of only minor encouragement or assistance;
- the suspect had sought to dissuade the victim from taking the course of action which resulted in their suicide;
- the actions of the suspect may be characterised as reluctant encouragement or assistance in the face of a determined wish on the part of the victim to commit suicide;
- the suspect reported the victim's suicide to the police and fully assisted them in their enquiries into the circumstances of the suicide or the attempt and his/her part in providing encouragement or assistance.

A constitutionally important decision in more recent years is that of Tony Nicklinson (see Case study 10.4), in which case the nine members of the Supreme Court deliberated over for six months. This case can be seen as indicating renewed moves to address changing the law on assisted suicide in the United Kingdom, with further considerations of the Human Rights Act 1998. Indeed, in this particular case, the Supreme Court viewed it as a domestic parliamentary decision to consider the position of assisted dying. Furthermore, in 2015, Parliament rejected another attempt to introduce a law for assisted dying (Marris, 2015), in which the Supreme Court referred to the DPP guidelines on decisions about prosecutions under Section 2

CASE STUDY 10.4	R (Nicklinson) v Ministry of Justice [2014] UKSC 38

Almost completely paralysed following a cerebrovascular accident ('stroke'), Tony Nicklinson (N) wanted to die, but his physical incapacity meant that he was unable to end his life other than through self-starvation. Therefore, he wished a doctor to assist with his suicide by injecting in him a lethal drug. Due to the unlawful nature of this request, he sought a declaration through the High Court for lawful termination of his life through the assistance of a doctor, and that the law preventing such was incompatible with Article 8 of the European Convention on Human Rights, which provides that everyone has the right to respect for private life, but that private life can be lawfully restricted for 'prevention of disorder or crime, for the protection of health or morals, or for the protection of rights and freedoms of others'. N died long before the Supreme Court gave its judgement in 2014; following his loss in the High Court, N declined all food and died of pneumonia. His wife continued to represent his case. The Court of Appeal followed by declining to grant N's declarations, followed by the Supreme Court majority decision to also decline the declarations, the counterargument to N's request being that legalising suicide be a 'slippery slope', and that criminalization was a necessary and proportionate way of protecting the rights and managing the risk of the vulnerable, the sick and the old who might otherwise be perceived as being pressured into availing themselves of assistance to end their lives.

of the Suicide Act 1961. Here, it was considered that flexibility was needed in the guidelines, whereby various relevant factors and the weights attached to such factors were to be considered individually in each case on its own merit.

Dignity and Dying

The term 'dying with dignity' is frequently used during debates and approaches to end-of-life issues; it was certainly conspicuous in the case of Tony Nicklinson. Article 5 of the European Court of Human Rights (ECtHR) and biomedicine makes patient consent obligatory for each health intervention, including the right to refuse treatment, as a way of respecting dignity and individual freedoms (Council of Europe, 1997). Horn and Kerasidou (2016) acknowledge that the interpretation of 'dignity' varies across countries. In England, it is mainly understood as respect for autonomy, based on the principle of bodily integrity; it is often associated with 'self-governance'. They further cite the Nuffield Council on Bioethics's (2002) earlier definition, which contends that an ingredient of human dignity is the 'presumption that one is a person whose actions, thoughts and concerns are worthy of intrinsic respect, because they have been chosen, organized and guided in a way which makes sense from a distinctively individual point of view'. The concept of dignity was also explored by Szawarski (2020), who declared '… yet though instinctively we think we know what it (*dignity*) means, we rarely pause to reflect on it'. Szawarski refers to the writings on morals by philosopher Immanuel Kant, who posited that 'the capacity for moral existence through autonomous exercise of will, that is rational thought… is the foundation of dignity'. Therefore, Kant viewed dignity as the 'respect or reverence that is required to acknowledge the capacity for reason and the moral conduct that is inherent to all rational beings' (Szawarski, 2020).

Tony Nicklinson exercised his own will by taking a course of action to starve himself to death, as he viewed his existence as 'dull', 'miserable', 'demeaning', 'undignified' and 'intolerable'. Although he exercised his autonomy, some could argue that his death was still undignified. Therefore, dying may create a situation in which dignity, being an innate part of a person's existence, means that their survival is threatened by a fear of losing capacity for rational thought. When caring for a terminally sick person, the nurse needs to be mindful of the changing reality of the patient, and that respect for the patient's dignity means demonstrating an awareness of how the patient's self-respect and rational thinking is ebbing away into a more vulnerable state of health.

Do Not Attempt Cardiopulmonary Resuscitation (DNACPR) Notices

In hospital and residential nursing care environments, where the patient has not made an advanced decision to refuse treatment, it is usually the lead clinician (i.e. consultant doctor) who makes a best interests decision as to whether a life-support machine should be switched off. In these instances, it is often the practice for the medical practitioner to place a 'do not resuscitate' (DNR) or DNACPR ('do not attempt cardiopulmonary resuscitation') instruction in the clinical records. In these instances, it is important for the nurse to discuss with the medical practitioner about the patient's prognosis so that they can understand the reasoning and ensure that the patient's relatives or carers have the same understanding. The case of *R (adult: medical treatment)* demonstrated the court supporting the reasoning behind a DNACPR notice, as cardio-pulmonary resuscitation (CPR) was unlikely to be successful. The Supreme Court recognised that there was no duty to provide treatment if it was futile to do so.

Two judgements which clarify the distinction between the duty *to provide* treatment and duty *not to provide futile* treatment include *R (Burke) v GMC* and *Aintree University Hospitals Foundation Trust v James*. In the case of *Burke*, the Court of Appeal held that once a patient is accepted into hospital, there is a positive duty to care for the patient in taking such steps to keep the patient alive; by contrast, in the Supreme Court ruling of *Aintree*, to consider the patient's treatment futile if it was not in the patient's best interests was deemed lawful, which confirmed the earlier judgement in *R (adult: medical treatment)*.

The British Medical Association, Resuscitation Council and Royal College of Nursing (2016) guidance upon CPR provides additional clarity with an aide-memoire which includes the following points:

> *...A CPR decision form, although not legally binding, should be regarded as an advance clinical assessment and decision and recorded to guide immediate decision-making in the event of a patient's cardiorespiratory arrest.*

> *The final decision whether or not to attempt CPR is clinically appropriate and lawful rests with the healthcare professionals responsible for the patient's immediate care at that time.*

> *When no explicit decision about CPR has been considered and recorded in advance, then there should be an initial presumption in favour of CPR.*

> *Decisions about CPR must be free from any discrimination, e.g. in respect of a disability.*

> *Clear and full documentation of decisions about CPR, the reasons for these, and the discussions that informed those decisions, is an essential part of high-quality care.*

> *When there is a clinical need for a DNACPR decision in a dying patient for whom CPR offers no realistic prospect of success, that decision should be made and explained to the patient and those close to the patient at the earliest and practicable and appropriate opportunity.*

> *When a patient or those close to a patient disagree with a DNACPR decision a second opinion should be sought.*

> *DNACPR does not override clinical judgement in the event of a reversible cause of the patient's respiratory or cardiac arrest, and is a best interests decision representative of a patient's disability, and must be guided by quality of life that the person themselves would be regarded as acceptable....*

End of life care for the terminally-ill patient is a potentially uncomfortable situation for a nurse, as they need to grapple with a number of emotions grounded upon their own perspectives, opinions and life experiences. As Taylor (2018) emphasizes, many nurses will have cared for patients for whom death represents a welcome end to intolerable pain and suffering. The views of the terminally-ill patient, and their family and health professionals may be that life-sustaining treatment is no longer in that patient's best interests; for 'nurses whose training and practice centre on the preservation of life, …some elements of end-of-life care may be counterintuitive, and nurses may find it difficult to put to one side their instinctive desire to do all they can to preserve life' (Taylor, 2018). Conversely, a diagnosis of terminal illness may be devastating news for a patient as 'the goal of expanded life vanishes' and in many cases, the patient's not unexpected deep suffering and depression can lead to their 'desire to hasten death' (Andorno and Baffone, 2014). Therefore, the nurse must be mindful of performing an essential role in providing compassionate care during the terminal stages of such a patient's life, even though the idea of discontinuing active life-sustaining treatment may be uncomfortable.

References

Academy of Medical Royal Colleges, 2008. A code of practice for the diagnosis and confirmation of death. Available at: https://aomrc.org.uk/.

Andorno, R, Baffone, C, 2014. Human rights and the moral obligation to alleviate suffering. In: Green, R, Palpant, N (Eds.), Suffering and bioethics. Oxford University Press, New York, pp. 182–200.

Brazier, M, Cave, E, 2016. Medicine, patients and the law, 6th ed. Manchester University Press, Manchester.

Baranzke, H, 2012. Sanctity-of-life' – a bioethical principle for a right to life? Ethical Theory and Moral Practice 15, 295–308.

British Medical Association, Resuscitation Council and Royal College of Nursing, 2016. Decisions relating to cardiopulmonary resuscitation: Guidance from the British Medical Association, the Resuscitation Council (UK) and the Royal College of Nursing. 3rd ed., 1st rev.

Chahal, 2009. Human rights: clarifying the law on assisted suicide. The Law Society Gazette. Available at: lawgazette.co.uk/law/human-rights-clarifying-the-law-on-assisted-suicide/52048-article.

Council of Europe, 1997. Convention for the protection of human rights and dignity of the human being with regard to the application of biology and medicine. Council of Europe, Strasbourg.

Crown Prosecution Service, 2021. Assisted suicide. Available at: https://www.cps.gov.uk/publication/assisted-suicide.

Director of Public Prosecutions, 2010. Suicide: policy for prosecutors in respect of cases of encouraging or assisting suicide (updated 2014). Available at: https://www.cps.gov.uk/legal-guidance/suicide-policy-prosecutors-respect-cases-encouraging-or-assisting-suicide.

Dworkin, R, 1994. Life's dominion: an argument about abortion, euthanasia, and individual freedom. Vintage Books, New York.

Frankena, WK, 1975. The ethics of respect for life. In: Barker, SF (Ed.), Respect for life in medicine, philosophy, and the law. John Hopkins University Press, Baltimore, pp. 24–62.

General Medical Council, 2020. Treatment and care towards the end of life: good practice in decision-making. Available at: https://www.gmc-uk-org/ethical-guidance/ethical-guidance-for-doctors/treatment-and-care-towards-the-end-of-life.

Herring, J, 2020. Medical law and ethics, 8th ed. Oxford University Press, Oxford.

Heywood, R, Mullock, A, 2016. The value of life in English law: revered but not sacred? Legal Studies 36 (4), 658–682.

Horn, R, Kerasidou, A, 2016. The concept of dignity and its use in end-of-life debate in England and France. Cambridge Quarterly of Healthcare Ethics 25, 404–413.

Kuhse, H, 1987. The sanctity of life doctrine in medicine: a critique. Clarendon, Oxford.

Leadership Alliance for the Care of Dying People, 2014. One chance to get it right: improving people's experience of care in the last few days and hours of life. Publication Gateway, London Reference 01509.

Marris R, 2015. Assisted Dying (No 2) Bill (HC Bill 7). Available at: www.parliament.uk.

Neuberger, J, 2013. More care, less pathway: independent review of the Liverpool care pathway. Department of Health.

Nuffield Council on Bioethics, 2002. Genetics and human behaviour: the ethical context. Nuffield Department of Bioethics.

Nursing and Midwifery Council, 2018. The Code: professional standards of practice and behaviour for nurses, midwives and nursing associates.

Oxford Dictionaries, 2018. Oxford dictionary of law, 9th ed. Oxford University Press, Oxford.

Szawarski, P, Kakar, V, 2012. Classic cases revisited: Anthony Bland and withdrawal of artificial nutrition and hydration in the UK. Journal of the Intensive Care Society 13 (2), 126–129.

Szawarski, P, 2020. Classic cases revisited – Tony Nicklinson and the question of dignity. Journal of the Intensive Care Society 21 (2), 174–178.

Taylor, H, 2018. Legal issues in end-of-life care 3: difficult decisions. Nursing Times 115 (1), 36–39.

CASES

- Aintree University Hospitals Foundation Trust (Respondent) v James (Apellant) [2013] UKSC 67
- Airedale NHS Trust v Bland [1993] AC 789
- An NHS Trust v DJ and others [2012] EWHC 3524 CoP
- B v An NHS Trust [2002] EWHC 429
- Pretty v United Kingdom [2002] 2 FLR 45
- R (Adult: Medical Treatment) (1996) 31 BMLR 127
- R (Burke) v GMC [2005] EWCA Civ 1003
- R (Nicklinson) v Ministry of Justice [2014] UKSC 38
- R (on the application of Purdy) v DPP [2009] UKHL 45
- Re A [1992] 3 Med LR 303
- W v M and others [2011] EWHC 2443

STATUTE

- Coroners and Justice Act 2009
- Human Rights Act 1998
- Suicide Act 1961

Contraception, Abortion and Sterilisation

KEY TERMS

Abortion
Contraception

Pro-life perspective
Sterilisation

Introduction

Abortion (also termed *termination of pregnancy*) and the regulation of pregnancy is a topic that arouses intense, passionate ethical and legal debate and conflict. There are those who regard abortion as the murder of an innocent living being, and those who claim that access to abortion is a fundamental human right and a central part of the campaign towards women's equality and autonomy. That is, a woman's decision should not be interfered with by medicine, religion or the law. Statistics provided by Public Health England (2018) show that 45% of pregnancies and one-third of the births in England were unplanned or associated with feelings of ambivalence. The Department of Health and Social Care (DHSC) statistics on abortion for 2019 showed a decline in abortion for women under the age of 18 over the last 10 years, particularly in the under-16 age group, from 4% to 1.4% per 1000 women. During the same period, the abortion rate for the 18–19 years age group decreased from 31.6% to 23.8% per 1000 women. However, there was an increase in the abortion rate for all ages 25 and over, with the largest increase in the 30–34 years age group, from 15.7% to 20.9% per 1000 women. What remained constant was marital status; 81% of the women having an abortion were single (DHSC, 2020). The law concerning these matters of abortion and fertility is succinctly described by Herring (2020) as seeking 'to strike a somewhat uneasy balance between recognising that the foetus has some interests; reinforcing medical control over pregnancy and birth control; and protecting the rights of the pregnant woman'.

Key Legislation

There are three major pieces of legislation that the nurse or midwife needs to be conversant with when caring for pregnant women:

Offences Against the Person Act 1861 protects children in utero by making abortion a criminal offence in England, Wales and Northern Ireland under Section 58 – where a woman is guilty of an offence if she unlawfully procures her own miscarriage; Section 59 – where it is an offence for any person who supplies drugs or instruments to be unlawfully used to procure abortion; Section 60 – where it is an offence for any person who secretly disposes of a child who died before, at, or after birth.

Infant Life (Preservation) Act 1929 in England and Wales. According to Section 1(1), any person who intends to destroy the life of a child capable of being born alive, by any wilful act that causes that child to die before it has an existence independent of its mother, is guilty of child destruction. Under Section 1(2), foetal viability is set at 28 weeks gestation, and evidence of such is *prima facie* (Latin: *accepted as correct until proved otherwise*) proof that she was, at the time, pregnant of a child capable of being born alive. This law is independently upheld in Northern Ireland via the Criminal Justice Act 1945.

Abortion Act 1967 (as amended by Section 37 of Human Fertilisation and Embryology Act 1990). Under Section 1(1), a person shall not be guilty of an offence when a pregnancy is terminated by a registered medical practitioner if two registered medical practitioners are 'of the opinion formed in good faith':

a. that the pregnancy has not exceeded its 24th week and that the continuance of the pregnancy would involve risk, greater than if the pregnancy were terminated, of injury to the physical or mental health of the pregnant woman or any existing children of her family; or

b. that the termination is necessary to prevent grave permanent injury to the physical or mental health of the pregnant woman; or,

c. that the continuance of the pregnancy would involve risk to the life of the pregnant woman, greater than if the pregnancy were terminated; or,

d. that there is a substantial risk that if the child were born, it would suffer from such physical or mental abnormalities as to be seriously handicapped.

The Abortion (Northern Ireland) Regulations 2020 provided new legislation in Northern Ireland from March 2020 that afforded women access to abortions up to 12 weeks, which was to be certified by a medical practitioner. Abortion beyond 12 weeks gestation was lawful in particular circumstances, such as when severe foetal impairment was present or when a fatal abnormality was detected in the foetus.

Contraception

Contraception was made readily available through the National Health Service (NHS) via the National Health Service (Family Planning) Act 1967. It enabled local health authorities to give advice to the wider population. Formerly, these services were limited to only those women whose health was at risk due to pregnancy. In recognition of a social problem, whereby low-income groups were more at risk of economic hardships by having more children than they could afford, a Private Members Bill was introduced in the House of Commons calling for the Parliament to respond to the issue of a rapidly growing population. Since the 1974 reorganisation of the NHS, family planning services were incorporated into the NHS with the supply of contraceptives and advice being issued free of charge with no restriction placed on the age and marital status of the person. Medical practitioners could then give contraceptive advice to a girl under the age of 16 without informing her parents, and had to seek her consent to inform her parents. However, this particular Department of Health and Social Security (DHSS) guideline on contraception that resulted in the high-profile campaign of parental control over teenage sexuality by Mrs Victoria Gillick (described in Chapter 9). Aside from the 'pill', other forms of female birth control, such as the intrauterine system (IUS) implants, patches and injections exist. However, the 'pill', introduced in 1961, remains a socio-medical and political issue that often divides opinion; this became the very issue that distinguished sexual activity from reproduction.

The Legality of Abortion

This chapter focuses specifically on induced (artificial) abortion.

Generally, if a pregnancy has not exceeded 24 weeks, and if two medical practitioners believe in 'good faith' that an abortion carries less risk to a woman's health (physical or mental) than continuing the pregnancy to term, it renders the abortion legal; this holds even when, in the eventuality, it would have been safer to continue the pregnancy to term, such as in a case where the abortion resulted in injury or death. Likewise, if a woman states that that she could not financially afford to continue the pregnancy, the medical practitioner is under no obligation to check whether she really is lacking in funds. Demonstrating that an opinion has been formed in good faith does not imply that authorising an abortion is 'right', but merely that the medical practitioner has not been dishonest or negligent in forming that opinion. Thus, a lawful abortion indicates that a medical opinion is based on facts that are lawful grounds for the termination of pregnancy. The 'good faith' opinion was created to reduce the number of illegal backstreet abortions as a consequence of unwanted pregnancies, as well as a disinclination to legislate an abortion on request. Since 1938, it has been established in law that an abortion is legal if a 'doctor' is 'of the opinion on reasonable grounds and with adequate knowledge of the probable consequences' that continuing the pregnancy would be physically or mentally harmful to the woman, and that risk assessment did not just extend to that concerning possible death. This consideration of the woman's mental and physical wellbeing was advanced through the Abortion Act 1967, indicating that an abortion was lawful 'if the continuance of the pregnancy would involve greater risk, greater than if the pregnancy were terminated, of injury to the physical or mental health of the pregnant woman'. In summary, any abortion carried out under Section 1(1)(a) of the Abortion Act 1967 – the grounds upon which the vast majority of abortions are carried out – would continue to be lawful provided the medical practitioners were acting in good faith, which was reliant on a sound base of medical evidence. Of international significance was the 1973 US Supreme Court case of *Roe v. Wade*, which ignited the debate concerning unduly restrictive state regulation of abortion. In *Roe v. Wade* the matter of abortion being criminalised in the majority of instances was viewed by many as a violation of a woman's constitutional right to privacy, guaranteed under the Fourteenth Amendment.

In the United Kingdom, McGuinness and Thomson (2015) noted that the Abortion Act 1967 was a 'compromise' concerning morals, political control of the procedure and seeking balance of interests of abortion-seeking women and foetuses. Furthermore, this was another political dimension of the tensions that existed regarding the control of the abortion process, namely between the Royal College of Obstetricians and Gynaecologists (RCOG) and Royal College of General Practitioners (RCGP). Although the NHS was viewed as the main provider of abortion services, its lack of preparation for the increasing number of abortions following the Act and lack of specific funding hindered progress as the work of hospital consultants increased (McGuinness and Thomson, 2015). Therefore, to improve the availability of abortion services alongside existing private sector provisions, the Abortion Law Reform Association (ALRA) planned to establish charitable bodies to help women seeking abortions. This independent sector has since become a necessary provider, and, as McGuinness and Thomson (2015) emphasises, has flourished and allowed women to circumvent 'obstructive physicians who wished to restrict the ability of women to access abortion services'.

According to Section 1 (2) of the Abortion Act 1967, it is legal to terminate a pregnancy because a woman's actual or foreseeable environmental, social or financial circumstances may be impacted due to continuing the pregnancy, or it impacts the woman's health. Thus, the law provides the medical practitioner the scope to decide who can have an abortion, stating that they may take into account a woman's environmental factors, but this is not an obligation. It is not always possible to separate the health effects of an abortion from a woman's wider socio-economic circumstances, such as her income, housing situation or family and services support network. Therefore, it is reasonable for a medical practitioner to consider these factors when determining whether to lawfully authorise an abortion. Setting a legal precedent for the protection of the woman's health was the early case of *R v Bourne*, where a doctor was acquitted for performing an abortion on a 14-year-old girl who had become pregnant as a result of rape. The court held that the pregnancy significantly threatened the girl's mental health, as she was presented as suicidal throughout and was considered to be in a life-threatening situation. Such circumstances are now covered by the emergency provisions of the Abortion Act (as amended).

Abortion is illegal if carried out for circumstances other than those permitted under the Abortion Act 1967. This includes the covert dispensing of miscarriage-inducing drugs to a pregnant woman – a crime under Section 58 of Offences Against the Person Act 1861 concerning administering poison or other noxious drugs. This covert approach was illustrated by intention in the case of *R v Ahmed*, where the husband of a non-English-speaking wife sought an abortion for her when she was 16–17 weeks pregnant. However, he had misrepresented his wife's wishes to the healthcare professionals, as she believed she was attending the clinic to have a minor operation to cure a problem with her blood. This misunderstanding raised concerns among the medical staff, and they sought a language interpreter from an Urdu-speaking nurse who clarified the issue; subsequently, the wife left her husband and had the child. It is also unlawful to carry out a gender-selective abortion based solely on the basis of parental preference of foetal gender. Where there are no health implications for the foetus or the woman, gender-selective abortion does not satisfy any of the grounds laid out in the Abortion Act 1967, and is thus unlawful [British Medical Association (BMA, 2020a)].

With such scope and discretion afforded to medical practitioners, it could incorrectly be assumed that in England and Wales, women can access abortion on request. That there is no right to abortion on the women's request is demonstrated in the following three ways:

- Lawfully, the decision to authorise an abortion lies with the judgement of two medical practitioners about the impact of abortion versus childbirth on the women's physical or mental health.
- The law does not stipulate that the medical practitioners 'must' take into account the woman's social circumstances.
- The Abortion Act 1967 allows medical practitioners the right to conscientious objection to performing or authorising an abortion, with the exception that it is necessary for life-saving purposes or to prevent severe, permanent injury to her health.

The government regulations provide for the completion of a certificate (Form HSA1) which deals with the medical practitioner's decision for the grounds for an abortion, and stipulates that such grounds for the abortion be specified in writing. However, there is no requirement for the medical practitioner to personally examine the woman. It is deemed to be good practice for a medical practitioner to rely on information provided by other members of the multi-disciplinary team in determining whether a woman meets the criteria for an abortion. The 1981 case of *Royal College of Nursing of the United Kingdom v. Department of Health and Social Security* established that abortion should be a procedure carried out in accordance with good practice, by a medical team consisting of midwives, nurses and allied health professionals as well as medical staff. The House of Lords ruled on appeal that the intention of the Abortion Act 1967 was to broaden the grounds on how lawful abortion can be obtained as part of ordinary medical care, and as such, nurses participating in pregnancy termination remain protected under the Act. This protection, however, stipulates that the physician (medical practitioner) who has prescribed the abortion

CASE STUDY 11.1	R (John Smeaton on behalf of SPUC) v The Secretary of State for Health [2002] 2 FCR 193

The Society for the Protection of Unborn Children (SPUC) sought for the courts to declare the supply of the 'morning-after' pill *Levonelle* a criminal offence under Sections 58 or 59 of the Offences Against the Persons Act 1861, purporting that it amounted to causing a 'miscarriage'. Together with the Abortion Act 1967, it was claimed that *Levonelle* was an abortifacient and not a contraceptive, and the Abortion Act procedures were thus not complied with. The claimant's (R) case was that any interference with a fertilised egg, if it led to the loss of that egg, was a procurement of a 'miscarriage' within the meaning of the 1861 Act, even if that interference occurred before the egg had implanted itself in the wall of the womb.

    The court rejected R's argument and dismissed his application, making it clear that a 'miscarriage' meant the termination of an established pregnancy and that there is no established pregnancy prior to implantation; therefore, there is no miscarriage if a fertilised egg is lost prior to implantation. The 'morning-after' pill was judged to be a form of contraception rather than an abortion. Additionally, current medical and lay understanding of the meaning of 'miscarriage' excludes results brought about by the contraceptive pill. Thus, there could be no miscarriage (or abortion) if there was no true carriage to the womb and the de-implantation of an egg. Furthermore, for the 'morning-after' pill to be effective, it has to be ingested no later than 72 hours post-coitus, when implantation, which would lead to pregnancy in the biological sense, would not have begun. The contraceptive pill operated before this time, and thus was not considered an abortifacient.

remain in charge and accept clinical responsibility throughout the procedure, even though they do not personally conduct every stage of the abortion.

    The case of *R (John Smeaton on behalf of SPUC) v The Secretary of State for Health* addressed the issue of whether the 'morning-after' pill – an emergency contraceptive – could be considered an abortifacient, which pertains to any drug/chemical that induces an abortion. In January 2001, the Prescription Only Medicines Act (Human Use) Amendment (No 3) Order 2000 came into force, whereby the emergency contraceptive Levonelle could be dispensed by pharmacists without a need for a medical prescription. The judgement in this case set the boundary between contraception and abortion, as detailed in Case study 11.1.

    This case did not concern pre- and post-conception, but rather the periods before and after implantation of the fertilised egg in the woman's womb. It also raised broader social and public health issues concerning the 'pill'. For example, if emergency contraception was not available, the number of abortions would greatly increase. Hypothetically, if the SPUC's argument was to be accepted, then use of the contraceptive pill, where it operated to prevent implantation (as opposed to conception), would be considered criminal. The question would then arise of unlawfulness with regard to millions of women using the 'pill'. It is also worth noting that the IUD (Intra-Uterine Device) is not an abortifacient but a form of contraception, as it acts as a spermicide rather than causing an abortion post-fertilisation.

    With respect to minors, under the Gillick principles, a person under the age of 16 who is not in local authority care, can consent to having an abortion. If there is a conflict between the rights of the minor (as the mother) and the parents' pressure on the daughter to have an abortion, a healthcare professional may take action to ensure that the Court decides on this matter under the Children Act 1989. For example, conflict between the pregnant minor and the parents may occur due to the minor being dependent on their help to house and bring up the child. For those below the age of 18, parents have the right to make decisions on 'best interests' grounds on behalf of the minor upon the premise that the (yet-to-be-born) child's welfare is the principal factor being considered. For pregnant females over the age of 16 who lack decision-making capacity, this situation falls under the Mental Capacity Act 2005.

Abortion – The 'Pro-Life' Perspective

Worldwide, abortion has become increasingly prevalent, and in many jurisdictions it remains a crime, although the restrictions and penalties for its contravention differ. The maternal rights (of the woman) versus the foetal rights (of the child) conflict. It is also noticeable that the law, social policy and medical practise sometimes treat a woman's interests in opposition to those of the foetus. For example, most religious leaders argue that the foetus (as a child in the womb) has a right to life and to the life they already possesses, and that no one should have the power to deny this right. Even within the medical profession, there are diverse views on abortion, where some professionals believe that the woman's desire is sufficient justification, but others object to abortion entirely on purely religious grounds. Many believe a foetus has the supreme right to life, and that the state is under an obligation to protect this right. Over the years, there has been a growing recognition of the personhood of an unborn child from both a medical and social perspective. This evolved the 'pro-life' movement, which supports the claims for both legal and ethical rights of the foetus, opposes the practise of abortion and takes the political stance that the foetus is a person with a right to life, and that at the time a woman becomes pregnant, she is carrying a new life. This stance is supported by numerous religious authorities, who believe that any action which deliberately destroys an embryo or a foetus is murder of a person, and is ethically and morally wrong.

Early commentary by Gillon (2001) describes the rationale for opposing abortion, that though the newly fertilised ovum and embryo does not have the attributes of a person – such as thinking, reflecting, imagining, experiencing or doing things for itself – the newly fertilised ovum and embryo has 'the future potential to do all those things… and therefore [must] be valued and respected for that potential and be accorded the same moral status and protection' that human beings accord each other. Furthermore, even though the embryo does 'not have the attributes of a person, such attributes are present in the genetic structure and organisation of the new human being, and left alone to develop, will gradually emerge' (Gillon, 2001).

From an ethical perspective of the 'sanctity of life', on the spectrum between individual cell and person, where then is the line drawn regarding when life becomes human? More importantly, what is a person (Robinson and Doody, 2022)? From the perspective of scientists and embryologists, there is a recognition that a new human being comes to be at fertilisation, and at the stage in which male and female chromosomes merge and the sex of the foetus is determined. The heart of the foetus commences beating at 18–25 days and from the 43rd day, electrical brain activity is recognised; consequently, at the time of the abortion, the foetus is arguably a defined human being (a life) that has existed from conception. Therefore, 'pro-life' advocates view abortion as a violation of a foetus's supreme right to live – akin to murder – and hold that the foetus has a right to be protected by the state.

Article 9 of the European Court of Human Rights (ECtHR) reinforced the freedom of thought, conscience and religion as one of the foundations of a democratic society. However, as Wicks (2009) notes, 'the right to manifest a religion or belief can be limited by the state… and prescribed by law for… public safety, public order, health and morals or the rights of others'. As with other medico-legal issues, Wicks (2009) raises the question of whether the state should be neutral between the religious beliefs of its citizens or if it should reflect some of these beliefs in encompassing a multicultural agenda. Although religious doctrine does not have a monopoly on the belief of sanctity of life, legislators should draw on both 'reason' and 'faith' when making decisions that impinge on other people's choices on how and even whether to reproduce (Wicks, 2009).

Conscientious Objection

Conscientious objection can be succinctly expressed as the choice to 'opt out' of engaging with a professional duty. As Dobrowolska et al. (2020) explains, this opting-out is solely because the action '…violates some deeply held moral or ethical value about right and wrong'. These values may exist before a person becomes a healthcare professional and may well have religious or other deep-rooted origins. Section 4 of the Abortion Act provides a conscientious objection clause, permitting medical practitioners to refuse to participate in abortion. However, this clause has an exception, in that it obliges medical practitioners to provide necessary treatment to save the life of, or 'prevent grave injury' to, a pregnant woman (BMA, 2020b). The General Medical Council (GMC, 2019) asserts that a doctor (medical practitioner) must inform patients of their right to see another doctor with whom they can discuss their situation, and provide the patients enough information to exercise that right. In providing this information, the doctor 'must not imply or express disapproval of the patient's lifestyle, choice or beliefs' (GMC, 2019). Section 4(1) of the Abortion Act allows for a nurse or midwife in England, Scotland and Wales to refuse to participate in the process of a treatment that results in the termination of a pregnancy because they have a conscientious objection; the same exceptions as those for medical practitioners, of saving life or preventing grave permanent injury, are applicable. Paragraph 4.4 of the nurse's Code (NMC, 2018) states that a nurse must inform their managers, colleagues and person receiving care that they have a conscientious objection to a particular procedure, such as abortion, and arrange for a qualified person to take over responsibility for the person's care. This issue of conscientious objection presents a complex ethical debate concerning clinical practitioners, and as Montgomery (2015) comments, who may be viewed as 'moral agents... to act freely and with integrity, following the dictates of their conscience'. Arguing against the statutory conscience clause of the Abortion Act, Montgomery states that conscientious objection relates to 'personal agency rather than professional identity', and that it serves to exempt professionals from considering the situation in which the patient finds themselves; the clinician's decision is based on matters unrelated to the patient's specific circumstances (Montgomery, 2015).

The Supreme Court judgement of *Doogan and Another v Greater Glasgow and Clyde Health Board* illustrates the broad spectrum of considerations regarding a conscientious objection to abortion. This case concerned an objection made by two senior midwives, where the conscientious objection clause was deemed to apply only to hands-on care and treatment of women in labour, and not to overseeing abortions performed by other midwives in the labour ward.

Sterilisation of Persons Lacking Capacity

The sterilisation of a 17-year-old minor with profound learning difficulties and a mental age of between 5–6 was addressed in the case of *Re B (A minor) (Wardship: Sterilisation)*. The minor was resident in a Local Authority care home, and although biologically sexually mature, she had no understanding of the link between sexual intercourse and pregnancy and was incapable of raising a child; her communication was also limited. She could not be relied upon to accept or take oral contraceptives, and it was planned that within two years, she would be transferred to an adult training centre where she would not receive the same level of daily care supervision. Accordingly, the House of Lords decided that in the 17-year-old's best interests, she should be sterilised; the minor's mother supported this decision. It is of note that the argument for the extra burden placed on the carers of a mentally ill or disabled woman, should she become pregnant, do not provide justifiable reasons for sterilisation. However, the court may consider an argument that the burden of supervising a non-sterilised woman may be so great that the care the woman is receiving could be adversely affected (*Re B [1987]*). This case set a precedent for all similar cases that come before the courts. From October 2007, consideration of whether a sterilisation was in the interests of a 17-year-old female would be presented before the Court of Protection. Children under the age of 16 would be heard under the Children Act 1989, as cases for the Family Division of the High Court.

The latter case of *Re A (Medical Treatment: Male Sterilisation)* concerning a 28-year-old man with Downs Syndrome whose mother wanted him to have a vasectomy, used the balance-sheet approach to make a best interests decision. This affirmed that sterilisation should be a last resort and that forcing sterilisation on incompetent persons, whether minors or adults, infringed on their rights under Articles 3 and 8 of the ECtHR. A contrasting outcome regarding the legal necessity of a vasectomy was made in *An NHS Trust v DE*, where the case of a 37-year-old man with learning disabilities and a mental age of 6–9 years was taken to the

Court of Appeal for a decision. The man, with good family, clinical and care worker support, was able to live partially independently and had developed a long-term relationship with a woman who also had a learning disability, albeit of a less severe nature. The woman had an unplanned pregnancy and gave birth to their child; with the man not wanting to have more children, his parents decided it would be in his best interests to have a vasectomy. Concerns over his lack of capacity were decided upon by the NHS Trust through further clinical assessments, which found that he had the capacity to consent to sexual intercourse, but not to using contraception. An independent psychiatric report concluded that a vasectomy was the most effective and beneficial course of action. The court, as per Article 8 of the ECtHR, Section 4(2) of the Mental Capacity Act and to maintain the man's semi-independent lifestyle, decided to grant this course of action.

F v West Berkshire Health Authority was a case regarding the lawfulness of a decision to sterilise a 35-year-old woman with a mental age of 5–6, who had permanently resided in a psychiatric hospital; she lacked the capacity to consent to the operation. She had entered into a sexual relationship with a fellow male patient, but her mother sought declaration from the court on the grounds that serious adverse consequences would result for her daughter should she go through with the pregnancy. The House of Lords granted the declaration, which was subsequently upheld by the Court of Appeal. This was a case of dilemma for the medical practitioner, in which if they did nothing, they would perhaps be deemed negligent; conversely, if they performed the operation, he could face a *prima facie* case of the tort of battery. The Court's decision was based on the medical professional acting in good faith and in the best interests of a patient who was incapable of giving consent.

However, this approach to best interests has received critical commentary in that 'F was the object of proceedings rather than the subject (a person)… as a clinical and legal dilemma to be resolved by others' (Jackson, 2018). From this perspective, the nurse as an observer of medical law and other court decisions may pause to consider whether the needs of the person/patient as the subject of such proceedings can become secondary to the debate and disputes that arise within the legal processes of decision-making.

In the Court of Appeal case of *Re S (Sterilisation: Patient's Best Interests)*, a 'best interests' application was made to carry out a hysterectomy on a 29-year-old woman (S), who had severe learning difficulties and was incapable of giving consent to medical treatment. S's mother and the medical practitioners had concerns about the risk of pregnancy as well as S's continuing heavy menstrual bleeding. The solicitor opposing the application argued that an alternative IUD would reduce the menstrual problems and provide adequate contraception, even though it would mean that S would have to undergo regular hospital visits for years to come, including IUD replacements. Alternatively, the judge regarded that it would be in S's best interests to undergo a subtotal hysterectomy, which would have the secondary effect of sterilisation as well as ending S's menstrual problems. The Court overturned the judge's decision on the grounds that less invasive alternatives should be tried first, and 'broader ethical, social, moral and welfare considerations' must be taken into account (Herring, 2020). In noting such considerations, more recent academic commentary has been critical of the MCAs list of relevant considerations, which gives no particular priority to a person's wishes (Jackson, 2018), and of the consideration and decisions made using the best-interests balance sheet approach (Coggan, 2016). In emphasising the importance of patient-centred law in medical decision-making for those who lack capacity, Coggan (2016) posits that there be a requirement where it is possible 'that equal weight be given to the wishes, feelings, beliefs and values of patients who have, and (to those) patients who are deemed to lack decision-making capacity'.

Unsuccessful Sterilisation

If a patient is sterilised in a defective way and has sexual intercourse which results in pregnancy, legal proceedings to recover damages could be brought against the medical practitioner if particular conditions were not met, as described by Varma and Gupta (2004). These include:

1. A gynaecologist's duty to inform women of the risk of failure and to carry out sterilisation in accordance with accepted good medical practice, and avoid foreseeable complications.
2. A duty of care, in which a claim for negligence may arise when the operation is not carried out in accordance with practices accepted as proper by a reasonable body of gynaecologists – the 'Bolam test'. This would include an omission of appropriate pre-operative counselling.
3. Avoiding a wrongful birth, where a negligent act would deprive the mother of a possibility to prevent the conception of a disabled child or have a lawful abortion.

The leading case of *McFarlane v Tayside Health Board* illustrates the complexity of bringing such negligence claims to the courts, as outlined in Case study 11.2.

CASE STUDY 11.2   McFarlane v Tayside Health Board [2000] 2 AC 59

Mr and Mrs McFarlane (Mr & Mrs M) were the parents of four children, and having decided to have no more children, Mr M underwent a vasectomy (male sterilisation) and was subsequently advised that contraception prevention was no longer necessary. However, Mrs M became pregnant. They sued the Health Board for the negligent advice. They made a claim for damages for the financial cost of raising the child and for Mrs M's discomfort and pain caused by pregnancy and childbirth. The claims were rejected by the court on the basis that pregnancy did not equate to the definition of physical injury, but was an associated result of conception; additionally, it held that the financial loss was surpassed by the benefits of parenthood. The Court of Appeal (Scotland) overturned the decision, and held that Mrs M was entitled to damages for the physical effects of pregnancy and birth, provided that negligence could be proved. The Court viewed unplanned conception as an infringement of Mr and Mrs M's right to family planning, and that there was a foreseeable consequence for which Mr and Mrs M could seek liability under the tort of negligence.

McFarlane acknowledged that women were entitled to recover general damages for pain and suffering during pregnancy and childbirth, and of loss of earnings during pregnancy. However, it held that the costs of raising a healthy child and a loss of earnings because of child-rearing responsibilities were not recoverable. By contrast, in *Rees v Darlington Memorial Hospital NHS Trust,* such costs were upheld, as the mother was disabled and considered to be in a position different from able-bodied parents.

References

British Medical Association (BMA), 2020a. The law and ethics of abortion: BMA views. September 2020 – post ARM update. Available at: https://www.bma.org.uk.

BMA, 2020b. The law and ethics of abortion. BMA views. September 2020. Available at: https://www.bma.org.uk.

Coggan, J, 2016. Mental capacity law, autonomy, and best interests: an argument for conceptual and practical clarity in the Court of Protection. Medical Law Review 24 (3), 396–414.

Department of Health and Social Care, 2020. Abortion statistics, England and Wales: 2019 Summary Information from the abortion notification forms returned to the Chief Medical officers of England and Wales: January to December 2019. Available at: https://www.gov.uk/dhsc.

Dobrowolska, B, McGonagle, I, Pilowska-Kozak, A, Kane, R, 2020. Conscientious object in nursing: regulations and practice in two European countries. Nursing Ethics 27 (1), 168–183.

General Medical Council, 2019. Good medical practice. Available at: https://www.gmc-uk.org/ethical-guidance/-for-doctors/personal-beliefs-and-medical-practices.

Gillon, R, 2001. Is there a 'new ethics of abortion'? Journal of Medical Ethics 27 (2), 5–9.

Herring, J, 2020. Medical law and ethics, 8th ed. Oxford university Press, Oxford.

Jackson, E, 2018. From 'doctor knows best' to dignity: placing adults who lack capacity at the centre of decisions about their medical treatment. Medical Law Review 81 (2), 247–281.

McGuinness, S, Thomson, M, 2015. Medicine and abortion law: complicating the reforming profession. Medical Law Review 23 (2), 177–199.

Montgomery, J, 2015. Conscientious objection: personal and professional ethics in the public square. Medical Law Review 23 (2), 200–220.

Public Health England, 2018. Guidance – health matters: reproductive health and pregnancy planning. Available at: https://www.gov.uk/government/publications/health-matters-reproductive-health-and-pregnancy-planning/health-matters-reproductive-health-and-pregnancy-planning.

Robinson, R, Doody, O, 2022. Nursing and Healthcare Ethics. Elsevier Ltd, Oxford.

Varma, R, Gupta, K, 2004. Failed sterilisation: evidence-based review and medico-legal ramifications. International Journal of Obstetrics and Gynaecology 111, 1322–1332.

Wicks, E, 2009. Religion, law and medicine: legislating on birth and death in a Christian state. Medical Law Review 17 (3), 410–437.

CASES

An NHS Trust v DE [2013] EWHC 2562 (Fam)
Doogan and Another v Greater Glasgow and Clyde Health Board [2014] UKSC 68.
F v West Berkshire Health Authority [1989] 2 All ER 545
McFarlane v Tayside Health Board [2000] 2 AC 59
R v Ahmed [2010] EWCA Crim 1949
R v Bourne [1938] 3 All ER 615
R (John Smeaton on behalf of SPUC) v The Secretary of State for Health [2002]
    2 FCR 193
Re A (Medical Treatment: Male Sterilisation) [2000] 1 FCR 193
Re B (A minor) (Wardship: Sterilisation) [1987] 2 All ER 206
Re S' (Sterilisation: Patient's Best Interests) [2000] 2 FLR 389
Rees v Darlington Memorial Hospital NHS Trust [2002] EWCA Civ 88
Roe v Wade (1973) 410 U.S. 113
Royal College of Nursing v DHSS [1981] 2 WLR 279

STATUTES

Abortion Act 1967 (as amended by Section 37 of Human Fertilisation and Embryology
    Act 1990)
Abortion (Northern Ireland) Regulations 2020
Children Act 1989
Infant Life (Preservation) Act 1929
Mental Capacity Act 2005
National Health Service (Family Planning) Act 1967
Offences Against the Person Act 1861
Prescription Only Medicines Act (Human Use) Amendment (No 3) Order 2000

Mental Ill-Health: Legal Aspects

KEY TERMS

Voluntary patient
Deprivation of Liberty
Compulsory admission

Holding powers
Guardianship
Discharge after-care

Introduction

Whereas the full extent and complexity of mental legislation is beyond the scope of this text, it is nevertheless important to understand the overall structure and application of the Mental Health Act (MHA) 1983. It is also beneficial for the nurse to grasp the essence of mental health legislation and its link with the Mental Capacity Act (MCA). This chapter focuses on adults requiring care; it does not deal with minors (under age of 18).

In England and Wales, the regulation of mental healthcare is governed by the MHA 1983 requirements, which was amended by the MHA 2007. The amended 2007 Act was directed at preventing discord between the MHA and the Human Rights Act (HRA) 1998; it is not a replacement but gives added protection (e.g. safeguards) to those vulnerable persons who come under the remit of health and social care. The MHA concerns the compulsory powers to detain (and treat) a person in hospital, when necessary. Law permits the detention and treatment of people who are mentally ill, including treatment being given to a competent person without their consent under particular circumstances, such as period of temporary incapacity that requires a 'best interests' decision; when there is a decline in their health status; for the protection of the general public from a dangerous mentally ill person; or to protect an individual from harming themselves. It cannot be presumed that persons with mental illness lack capacity, as the case of *Re' C (Adult Refusal of Treatment)* illustrated.

As it stands, the MHA can present as vast and complex, and it is advisable for the clinical practitioner to refer to the Code of Practice (Department of Health, 2015) which has an operational focus. Also, a more concise, easy to read guide by Barber et al. (2017) provides relevant background as well as detailing all aspects of MHA 1983 including the 2007 revisions.

The Voluntary Patient

Herring (2020) states that the issue of detaining the dangerous mentally ill person dominates the law in mental health and 'creates a skewed vision of mental illness in our society'. Recognising the presence of adverse, unconstructive attitude towards mental illness in society, Herring further emphasises that in the vast majority of the cases, mental illness is treated voluntarily in the community with no special legal regulation, and perhaps even 'a larger amount goes unrecognised and untreated' (Herring, 2020).

Before studying the key parts of the MHA, it is essential to understand the person who is admitted informally to hospital – the voluntary patient. When a patient needs to be admitted to a hospital for treatment for mental disorder, admission should be achieved without resorting to compulsory detention under the MHA, unless the use of such compulsion is necessary. This implies that either the patient consents to admission, if capable of so doing, or that it is in their best interests under Section 5 of the MCA, 2005, when they lack capacity. In contrast to a patient detained under the MHA, in theory, an informal patient consents and has no objection to their admission to or treatment at a hospital, and thus, may leave the hospital at any time. However, there are some concerns in situations when the patient lacks capacity and is unable to express their desire to leave or not be treated, but has nowhere to go and no person to advocate on their behalf. This was highlighted in the *Bournewood* case (see Chapter 2), where the leading judgment identified two categories of persons to whom Section 131 (informal admission of patients) of the MHA provisions applied: (i) those who enter hospital as in-patients who have the capacity to consent to such an admission – voluntary; (ii) those who, through a lack of capacity to consent, do not object (as in *Bournewood*), described as 'informal' patients. However, on account of their informal status, such patients do not have protection under the provisions of the Mental Health Review Tribunal (MHRT); therefore, when this minority group of 'de-facto' passive informal patients wish to leave hospital or their carers decide to ask for their discharge even as their psychiatrists refuse, they cannot appeal to the MHRT.

Case study 12.1 of *Re C (An Adult: Refusal of Medical Treatment)* illustrates how a mentally ill person can still retain capacity to understand information and exercise their right to decide on their medical treatment and care.

CASE STUDY 12.1	**Re C (An Adult: Refusal of Medical Treatment) [1994] 1 All Er 819**

C was a long-term formally detained patient in a psychiatric hospital who suffered from paranoid schizophrenia. After developing gangrene in one leg, he received medical advice that his leg needed a below-the-knee amputation, as he had only a 15% chance of survival without the surgery. C repeatedly refused to consent to the amputation, stating that he would rather die with two legs than live with one, and, amidst particular delusional beliefs, that God would save him. Thus, C sought an injunction restraining the hospital from amputation without his express consent. The hospital asserted that C's capacity to give a conclusive decision had been impaired by his mental illness and that he had failed to grasp the risk of death if the operation was not conducted. The question was whether it had been established that his capacity has been so reduced by his chronic mental illness that he did not sufficiently understand the nature, purpose and effects of the surgical treatment offered. This depended on whether he understood and recollected information as to the advised treatment, had believed this information and had estimated it when making a choice.

The court found that although C's capacity to make a decision had been compromised by his mental illness, there was no evidence that he lacked sufficient understanding of the nature, purpose and effects of the advised surgery. Indeed, it appeared that C had understood, retained and believed the relevant treatment information, and had arrived at a clear decision. Therefore, he had exercised his right to self-determination, as he was capable of giving or refusing consent. Hence, that C had a mental illness was irrelevant, as a person must be presumed to have capacity regardless of their underlying circumstances, and the capacity test was related to his ability to make the specific decision and not his overall position.

Deprivation of Liberty Safeguards

The MCA Deprivation of Liberty Safeguards (DoLS) were introduced in 2009 via the MHA 2007 amendments. Pertaining to persons in psychiatric and general hospitals as well as care homes, they were introduced in response to the European Court of Human Rights (ECtHR) judgement in the case of *HL v UK* (also known as *Bournewood*), which concluded that common law, which had been widely used to hold and treat patients lacking capacity, was inadequate to satisfy the European Convention of European Rights (ECHR) with regard to Article 5. However, at the time of its introduction, the new legislation was criticised for its unclear interface with the existing MH law. The DoLS were introduced to run parallelly with the MHA; however, as Cairns et al. (2010) point out, 'the MCA and MHA are grounded in very different principles... – patient autonomy and best interests v. Paternalism and risk reduction – there is significant overlap in coverage of the two statutes'. Principally, nurses should recognise that the MCA relates to a person's functioning – that is, their capacity (or incapacity) to make a particular decision – whereas the MHA relates to a person's status as someone diagnosed as having a mental disorder, within the meaning of the MHA and subject to its powers.

The 2006 case of *JE v DE* emphasised the lack of clarity regarding patient autonomy and deprivation of liberty (See Case study 12.2).

CASE STUDY 12.2	JE v DE and Surrey County Council and Others [2006] EWHC 3459 (Fam)

The case of JE v DE highlighted early difficulties in identifying what constituted a deprivation of liberty, concerning a 76-year-old man (DE) who was blind and memory impaired following a Cerebro-Vascular Accident (a stroke), and suffered from dementia. The evidence strongly suggested that he lacked capacity. His wife (JE) claimed she could no longer care for him and protested against the council's lack of support in caring for him by 'putting him on the streets'. He was subsequently accommodated by the County Council. Whilst in accommodation, although he never tried to leave, he repeatedly indicated that he wanted to return home and live with his wife. The County Council advised his wife not to attempt to take him home as they thought it was not in his best interests. However, having made her point, JE challenged this situation and desired for him to return home. She claimed this was a deprivation of his liberty and a breach of his human rights under Article 5, as a person could also be effectively deprived of their liberty by the misuse of locked doors as physical barriers. The Court concluded that this was a deprivation of DE's liberty on the fundamental grounds that he was under the control of the County Council, and thus deprived of his liberty to leave the accommodation, in the sense of being able to remove himself permanently and live with whom he chose.

Other notable court cases that demonstrate the context of deprivation of liberty include *G v E v A Local Authority v F* and *London Borough of Hillingdon v Neary*.

A later 2014 Supreme Court decision of *P v Cheshire West and Chester Council; P and Q v Surrey County Council* followed two previous Court of Appeal decisions, which redefined what constituted a deprivation of liberty as opposed to a restriction of movement. Consequently, an 'acid test' was suggested to assess whether a person is deprived of their liberty, namely, 'whether they are subject to continuous supervision and control and not free to leave'; this is not to be equated with simply testing whether the person is free to leave.

The DoLS provide legal protection for those vulnerable people who are, or may become, deprived of their liberty, within the meaning of Article 5, in a hospital or care home (registered under the Care Standards Act 2000), placed either under public or private measures. However, they do not apply to people detained under the MHA. Thus, DoLS seek to protect those whose circumstances create a deprivation of liberty that appears unavoidable, but is in their own best interests.

In principle, every effort should be made by commissioners and healthcare providers to prevent deprivation of liberty; however, if unpreventable, it should be for no longer than is required. The safeguards provide for deprivation of liberty to be made legal through authorisation processes that are intended to prevent subjective decisions to deprive a person of liberty and give the right to challenge DoLS authorisations. Additionally, these safeguards imply that a 'managing authority' (i.e. relevant hospital or care home) must seek authorisation from a 'supervisory body' (e.g. primary care trust; a Local Authority or a local health board; or the Welsh Assembly) to be legally able to deprive a person of their liberty. There are two types of authorisation – standard and urgent. Standard is for up to a year involving individual assessors and authorised by the supervisory body. The assessment process requires that the views of the person concerned and their family and friends be taken into account, and that the consideration of the least restrictive options for care be considered. Urgent is for 7 days and is authorised by the hospital or care home themselves; it can be extended up to 14 days with permission from the supervisory body. Prior to such authorisations, the supervisory body must be satisfied that the person has a mental disorder and lacks capacity to decide about their residence or treatment. A decision as to whether deprivation of liberty occurs depends on the context and conditions of each case; it is not necessary or correct to apply for a deprivation of liberty authorisation for each person who is in a hospital or care home, simply because they lack capacity to decide whether they should be there. A nurse must ensure that such patients within their care are protected by the safeguards, and in particular, the periodic independent check of whether the arrangements for the care and treatment of such persons are in their best interests.

DoLS Assessment

To give a standard authorisation of a deprivation of liberty, six assessments must be undertaken: age, mental health, no refusals, mental capacity, eligibility and best interests. This is detailed within the Mental Capacity Act Deprivation of Liberty Safeguards Code of Practice (Ministry of Justice, 2008). Registered nurses are among the group of health and social care professionals that can undertake these assessments, with the exception of the mental health assessment.

The purpose of the *age assessment* is to confirm whether the relevant person is aged 18 or over, and the *no refusals assessment* is to establish that an authorisation to deprive the relevant person of their liberty does not conflict with another existing authority for decision-making for that person. For example, if the relevant person has made an advance decision to refuse treatment that remains in force and is applicable to some or all of the treatment that is the purpose for which the authorisation is requested, then a standard authorisation cannot be given. The purpose of the *mental capacity assessment* is to establish whether the relevant person lacks capacity to decide whether they should be accommodated in the relevant hospital or care home to be cared for or treated. Carried out by a best interests assessor, it refers to the relevant person's capacity to make this decision at the time of need. The starting assumption is always that a person has the capacity to make the decision. The *mental health assessment* is to establish whether the relevant person has a mental disorder (i.e. is of 'unsound mind'), as defined by the MHA 1983. This is necessary to meet the requirements of Article 5 (1), and includes those with a learning disability but excludes those solely with dependence on alcohol or drugs. This assessment must be carried out by a registered medical practitioner, approved under Section 12 of the MHA, or a registered medical practitioner who possesses at least three years post-qualifying experience in the diagnosis and treatment of mental disorders. It is worth noting that any

doctor undertaking a mental health assessment cannot be a best interests assessor. The *mental capacity assessment* establishes whether the relevant person lacks
the capacity to decide whether they should be hospitalised or provided accommodation in a care home for treatment or health/social care. The assumption is
always that a person has the capacity to make the decision, and the assessment
refers to a person's decision-making capacity at the time of need. The *eligibility
assessment* considers the person's status with respect to the MHA; that is, a person
subject to most forms of detention under the MHA is not eligible for DoLS, or
if there is an obligation placed upon them under the MHA, such as a requirement to reside somewhere else; a guardianship order; s17a supervised community
treatment or a Section 17 'leave of absence'. As with the mental capacity assessment, in England, this undertaking must be by an assessor who is eligible to
carry out either a mental health or best interests assessment, but the regulation
does not apply to Wales. The purpose of the *best interests assessment* is to establish
whether a relevant person is being deprived of their liberty, and if so, whether it
is in their best interests and is both necessary to prevent harm and proportionate
to the likelihood of the person suffering harm and the seriousness of such harm.
As with other assessments under the MCA, the best interests assessor should
seek the opinions of those interested in the care and welfare of the person, such
as close relatives, carers or advocates working with the person. If the best interests
assessment supports deprivation of liberty, the assessor must state the authorisation period up to a maximum of 12 months.

In July 2018, the government published a Mental Capacity (Amendment) Bill,
under which DoLS will be replaced by Liberty Protection Safeguards (LPS), which
will see a streamlining of the DoLS authorisation process. This passed into law in
2019 and is scheduled for implementation in April 2022. In contrast with DoLS,
which can only be used to protect a person's rights if they are aged 18 or over and
are being cared for in a hospital or care home, the LPS will apply to everyone age
16 or over who is being cared for in any setting, such as supported living or in their
own home with carers.

Compulsory Admission and Detention Under MHA

Section 2 – Admission to Hospital for Assessment

Section 2 provides for the admission and detention of a patient for the purposes of
assessment (and, where appropriate, treatment) for up to 28 days. The grounds for
admission are:

  a. the patient must be suffering from some form of mental disorder at the time
     of the application;
  b. the mental disorder must be of a nature or degree to warrant their detention in
     hospital for assessment/assessment followed by medical treatment, and must
     be in the interests of the patient's own health or safety, or with a view for the
     protection of others.

c. 'Protection of others' is understood to mean protection from both physical and serious psychological harm. Thus, the nature, likelihood and level of risk from which others are entitled to protection must be considered before an application for compulsory admission is made.

The purpose of the admission is to assess the patient's health condition, identify the form(s) of disorder from which they are suffering and to treat such. Applications for such an admission are usually made by an Approved Mental Health Professional (AMHP); however, in some cases, these are made by the patient's nearest relative. An AMHP is a specially trained professional authorised by a local authority, such as a registered nurse or social worker, who has the statutory responsibility to coordinate an assessment of a person, ensuring that when detained under the MHA, the person is aware of their rights and is dealt with under the least restrictive principle. The AMHP has a number of specific duties, including: interviewing the patient 'in a suitable manner' prior to the application; satisfying that they have taken into account the wishes expressed by the patient's relatives; and/or considered any other relevant circumstances necessary for the application. In addition to the information the AMHP is required to give to the nearest relative, wherever possible, the professional should ascertain the views of the nearest relative about their own needs as well as of the patient's. It is essential that they inform the nearest relative of the reasoning behind the application for admission and the potential effects of such an application.

The formal and legal process of making the application requires the AMHP to receive two medical recommendations, one of which should be from a Section 12 approved registered medical practitioner, i.e. consultant psychiatrist or general practitioner - one of which (if practicable) have had a previous acquaintance with the patient. A Section 12 medical practitioner must 'personally examine the patient' before completing the medical recommendation. No more than 5 days are allowed to elapse between the two examinations. If direct access to the patient is not immediately possible (e.g. locked entry to patient's residence) and there is a postponement of an examination to negotiate access, then the police may be allowed to exercise their lawful power of entry. Once the application has been 'duly completed', the applicant has the authority to convey the patient to a hospital or authorise the police or ambulance service to do the same. This must occur within 14 days from the last medical examination. The 28-day detention period commences when the admission documents are received by the hospital managers.

On admission, the hospital managers have a duty to ensure that the patient understands the effect of compulsory detention and of the scope of the section of the MHA they have been detained under. When a person is admitted under Section 2 and the assessment indicates that they need treatment exceeding the permitted 28 days, then application for detention under Section 3 should be made at the earliest. It is not possible to renew an application for admission under Section 2 or for there to be a 'back to back' application.

Section 3 – Admission to Hospital for Treatment

Many provisions relating to applications under Section 2 also apply to an application under Section 3, which lasts for 6 months and can thereafter be renewed. The application can be made by either the patient's nearest relative or an AMHP with the requirement for examination by two doctors as defined under Section 2. There are three grounds for admission which are subject to the opinion of a medical doctor, that:

a. The person is suffering from mental disorder of a nature or degree which makes it appropriate for them to receive medical treatment in a hospital. The MHA defines mental disorder as 'any disorder or disability of the mind', but it is unsatisfactory to merely indicate that a person has a mental disorder. Therefore, the disorder must be such that it cannot be treated in the community, even though there is no need to identify exactly from what disorder the person is suffering.

b. It is necessary for the health or safety of the patient and/or for the protection of others that the patient receive such treatment, and it can only be provided if they are detained under Section 3. As with Section 2, a person can be detained if they are a danger to self or others. If the patient is competent and able to consent to treatment, then there is no requirement to detain.

c. Appropriate medical treatment is available to the patient. This may appear misleading (i.e. not stating mental illness or psychiatric), but any reference in the MHA to medical treatment in relation to mental disorder shall be '…construed as a reference to medical treatment the purpose of which is to alleviate, or prevent a worsening of, the disorder or one or more of its symptoms or manifestations' (Herring, 2020). Under Section 145 following the 2007 amendments concerning treatment, this includes nursing, psychological intervention and specialist mental health rehabilitation.

If the patient is competent and refuses treatment, then the treatment cannot be imposed upon them, except under Section 63 of the MHA; this section permits treatment for mental disorder but does not authorise treatment for physical conditions unrelated to the mental disorder. Historically, this distinction has been challenged in respect of the broad interpretations concerning treatment of a mental health condition. The following cases expand on the dilemmas these interpretations can present: *Norfolk and Norwich Healthcare (NHS) Trust v W*, concerning the detention of an elderly person with limited mental capacity; *Re KB (Adult) (Mental Patient: Medical Treatment)* concerning anorexia nervosa; *B v Croydon Health Authority* concerning forced feeding and personality disorder; *Tameside and Glossop Acute services Trust v CH* concerning caesarean section for a psychotic person; and *Nottinghamshire Healthcare NHS Trust v RC* concerning blood transfusion for a Jehovah's witness with a personality disorder.

Section 4 – Emergency Admission

This is essentially an admission under Section 2, but under circumstances where there is an 'urgent necessity' and insufficient time to obtain a second medical recommendation. The patient may be admitted for up to 72 hours, after which the application ceases to have effect. The 72-hour period commences from the time the person is admitted to the hospital. The patient must be admitted within 24 hours from the time they were medically examined or the application was made, whichever is earlier.

During this time, attaining a second recommendation will convert Section 4 into Section 2, and the patient may be detained for the remainder of the 28-day period. The grounds for admission are for the purpose of assessment, as laid down in Section 2, with an application made by an AMHP or the nearest relative; however, unlike Sections 2 or 3, the applicant must have seen the patient in the previous 24 hours. Furthermore, unlike Section 2, the medical practitioner need not be a specialist (Section 12) doctor, although, if practical, should be a doctor who knew the patient previously.

At the end of the 72-hour period the patient is free to leave unless another route of compulsory admission is invoked; the MHA does not permit a renewal of the detention. Therefore, if the patient is to remain detained, then the application must either be converted to a Section 2 (with a written second medical recommendation) or Section 3 application. Notably, a conversion to Section 2 for a period of 28 days is from the date of admission under Section 4; however, a medical recommendation under Section 4 cannot be used to support a following application under Section 3.

Sections 135 and 136

Section 135 provides for a magistrate to issue a warrant authorising a police officer to enter premises, using force if necessary, and is the only provision of the MHA which permits such access; though, powers of entry can also come from criminal law. Section 135(1) provides a power of entry and power to remove a person to a place of safety for up to 72 hours, when there are concerns about them, and it is deemed necessary that they be assessed, and when access cannot be otherwise gained. Section 135(1) allows for an AMHP to give information under oath that there is reasonable cause to suspect a person is suffering from a mental disorder; has been or is being, ill-treated, neglected or kept otherwise than under proper control in any place within the jurisdiction of the justice; or is unable to care for themselves and is living alone in any such place. The warrant provides for entry and, 'if thought fit', the removal of a person to a 'place of safety' with a view to making an application for them under the MHA or other arrangements for treatment/care. Compulsory treatment provisions do not apply to any person detained until such arrangements have formally been made.

Section 135(2) allows for a police officer or other authorised person to give information under oath regarding a person liable to be detained, such as a patient subject to compulsory detention under the MHA and/or has gone absent without permission of leave (AWOL). The warrant provides authority for entry and removal of the person when there is reasonable cause to believe that they will be found on the premises, but within the jurisdiction of justice and where admission to such premises has been refused. The person is then subject to being returned to the place of safety under the MHA, which can include local authority accommodation, hospitals, police stations and 'any other suitable place'.

Section 136 gives police officers power to remove a person from a public place to a 'place of safety'. This removal is for up to 72 hours to enable examination by a doctor and interview by an AMHP to make any necessary arrangements for treatment or care. As with Section 135, compulsory treatment provisions do not apply. Upon effecting Section 136, the police officer must judge as to whether the person is suffering 'from mental disorder and to be in immediate need of care or control' and thinks it necessary to remove the person to a 'place of safety' in the person's interests or for the protection of others. Although an A&E Department may be deemed a place of public access, a hospital ward is not. Furthermore, though the 'place of safety' has the same meaning as in Section 135, the MHA code advises that it is generally not preferable for a 'place of safety' to be a police station, and that an identified place of safety is under no obligation to take the person in. However, under the MHA 2007, there is provision for the person to be transferred from one place of safety to another. Under particular circumstances, the use of physical force (e.g. restraint) may be required when removing a person, or within a place of safety, to prevent harm to the person themselves or others; this should be proportionate to the risk of harm if restraint was not used and be of the least restrictive method.

Section 136 has historically proved challenging for the police and healthcare professionals to implement. Viewed as a 'difficult and complex' piece of legislation, there are differences in the levels of knowledge and perceptions of the section, as well as interpretations and professional responsibilities at an operational level between police and clinical staff (Lynch et al., 2002). More recently, Lord Adebowale chaired an enquiry (Adebowale, 2013) conducting research within the Metropolitan Police service which evidenced the misunderstandings that continued to exist regarding Sections 136 and 135, and when or whether MHA powers should be used; this included differing perceptions on the 'place of safety'. The report made a number of recommendations, a key theme of which was the need for more effective joint-working, protocols and guidelines to provide effective and better coordinated services to vulnerable persons with mental health issues.

Local authorities, NHS commissioners, hospital trusts, police forces and ambulance services should have local arrangements (Mental Health Partnership Boards) in place to ensure that those experiencing acute mental health problems are able to access the most appropriate specialist provider for assessment and care. Such multi-agency arrangements should include a local policy overseeing all aspects of practice concerning Sections 135 and 136.

The Human Rights Act (HRA) has also occasioned much consideration and critical debate regarding the restrictions placed upon a person's liberty by the MHA. The following case of *M.S. v UK* (Case study 12.3) is an example of a decision made by the ECtHR which addresses a dilemma between the MHA and a person's right to liberty.

Section 5 – Doctors and Nurses Holding Powers

Section 5 concerns powers to 'hold' an in-patient who, at the time, is not liable to detention under the MHA. Its purpose is to prevent the patient from leaving the

CASE STUDY 12.3	**MS v UK 24527/08 [2012] ECtHR 804**

After having assaulted his aunt, MS was taken to a police station under Section 136 of the Mental Health Act; however, the Forensic Medical Examiner assessed him as not fit for interview, and the local psychiatric intensive care unit refused to admit him on the grounds that he required forensic secure accommodation. Consequently, there was a delay in transferring him there. This delay led to detention beyond the 72-hour limit under Section 136, and MS made a claim for negligence and breach of his human rights under Article 3. Following dismissal of the case in the domestic courts, the case proceeded to the European Court of Human Rights, which did not criticise of the initial detention in a police station under Section 136 (i.e. his physical and nutritional needs), but did conclude that MS was in a state of considerable vulnerability throughout the detention, which had required him to have appropriate psychiatric treatment. It was ruled that the conditions that MS endured were an affront to human dignity and had reached the threshold of degrading treatment for the purposes of Article 3. MS was awarded compensation for damages.

hospital whilst an application for assessment or admission for treatment is being considered. The 'holding' power can also be exercised with respect to a patient receiving treatment for a physical illness in an acute hospital, but not as an out-patient attending the A&E Department.

Section 5(2) concerns a registered medical practitioner or the approved clinician (AC) in charge of a patient's treatment, to prevent an in-patient from leaving the hospital. This holding power can last up to 72 hours to enable an application for detention. The registered medical practitioner or AC must examine the patient and make an application, having provided a written report to the hospital managers, which provides the authority to detain. This 72-hour period cannot be renewed, extended, or prolonged past its expiry. Additionally, the registered medical practitioner or AC may nominate another member of staff within the hospital to act as a nominated deputy. Where the in-patient is receiving both psychiatric and medical treatment, the Consultant Psychiatrist is the 'doctor in charge of treatment'; if the registered medical practitioner 'holding' the patient is not a psychiatrist, then they are required to make immediate contact with one. If a patient detained under Section 5(2) requires transfer to another provider hospital, then an application under Section 2 or 3 should be made as soon as possible and addressed to the receiving managers of the other in-patient unit before the patient is admitted to the new provider.

Section 5(4) gives registered nurses the power to detain a patient for up to 6 hours. Usually, it is applied in situations where a registered medical practitioner is not immediately available to exercise their powers under Section 5(2). It is the personal decision of the nurse to exercise this power, and thus they cannot be ordered to exercise it. Essentially, Section 5(4) provides a short period of detention to allow the medical practitioner to come to the ward. This power is not renewable and is only exercised whilst the patient is on hospital premises. Once the medical practitioner arrives, they must decide whether to 'convert' the 5(4) into 5(2), upon which the patient may be detained for the remainder of the 72-hour period. The nurse must deem that the patient 'is suffering from a mental disorder to such a degree that it is necessary for his own health and safety or for the protection of others for him to be immediately restrained from leaving the hospital…'. The exercise of this power only pertains to an in-patient receiving treatment for a mental disorder. The holding power of section 5(4) lapses on the arrival of a registered medical practitioner, with the 6-hour period being counted as part of the 72-hour period, should Section 5(2) be applied.

Guardianship

Under Section 7 of the MHA, a person subject to a guardianship order will have a named guardian, usually a Local Social Services Authority (LSSA)-appointed worker or a private individual named by the LSSA. Guardianship provides an alternative to detention for compulsory treatment by requiring a person who is 16 years or older with a mental disorder to: reside at an address specified by the guardian; attend any place specified by the guardian at a specified time for medical treatment, occupation, education or training; and allow access to their place of residence to any person named by the guardian, such as a doctor or AMHP. Two medical recommendations are required, as is an application by the AMHP or the person's nearest relative for 'Guardianship' grounds to be met. It is for a period of 6 months, renewable for a further 6 months and thereafter on a yearly basis. Under guardianship, no treatment may be given to the patient without their consent on the grounds that the patient is suffering from a mental disorder of a nature or degree that warrants guardianship and is necessary in the interests of the welfare of the patient or for the protection of others.

Discharge from Hospital After Care: Section 117 and Community Treatment Orders

Section 117 of the MHA provides that patients detained under the Act have a right to aftercare as a duty provided by the health and social care services, which must provide any aftercare that they consider necessary. This aftercare should continue for as long as the health and social services consider it necessary; the decision to end aftercare should be a joint-agency one. Aftercare plans are the duty of the Responsible Clinician (RC), who should take the lead in establishing a care plan and organising the management of the patient's continuing care needs, considering the multidisciplinary approach and wishes and needs of the patient and their relatives/friends. The RC is usually a Consultant Psychiatrist, but since 2007, a registered nurse can also be an RC. In the *Clunis v Camden & Islington* Court of Appeal judgement, aftercare services were stated as including '…social work, support in helping the ex-patient with problems of employment, accommodation or family relationships, the provision of domiciliary services, and the use of day centre and residential facilities'. Even though this aftercare is a duty of provision, there is no element of compulsion under Section 117; therefore, a patient cannot be made to accept such services. Nevertheless, if a patient absents themselves from the place of residence required in the guardianship application, they can be taken into custody and returned accordingly to the place of residence by a police officer or a specified person.

Section 17a Community Treatment Orders

Introduced into English and Welsh legislation by the MHA 2007, the Community Treatment Orders (CTOs) are applied to a patient already subject to Section 3 and certain other sections of the MHA, and liable to be detained for treatment. The CTO is intended to allow suitable patients to be safely treated in the community rather than in a hospital. The RC, in agreement with the AMHP, can implement a CTO, which has the same time period as a Section 3 detention – a maximum of 6 months, subject to a renewal for 6 months and thereafter for 12-month periods. The CTO establishes the terms under which a person must accept treatment and specialist mental health services whilst living in the community. These can include medication, psychotherapy/counselling, multi-disciplinary monitoring, care and rehabilitation. Mandatory and discretionary conditions attached to a CTO are as follows:

- Mandatory: The patient must make themselves available for examination by the RC if the CTO is going to be renewed, as well as for examination by the Second Opinion Appointed Doctor (SOAD) if requested to do so for consenting to certain treatment conditions.
- Discretionary: In agreement with the AMHP, specify necessary conditions to ensure that the patient receives medical treatment or prevent the patient from being at risk of harm and protect others who may be at risk from the patient.

The CTO patient may be recalled to hospital and detained for 72 hours, during which time they will be subject to the compulsory treatment conditions. Additionally, the order can be revoked.

Recent evidence has shown that CTOs are often viewed by the patients as coercive and restrictive (Department of Health and Social Care, 2018). Thus, the future use of CTOs has been reviewed and is subject to reform, following a final independent review report in December 2018. A number of recommendations were made, including addressing the longstanding issue of over-representation of Black, Asian and minority ethnic (BAME) groups among those detained under the MHA, which, over recent years, has been revealed through the use of CTOs.

For nurses involved in the clinical decision-making process of persons being considered for care and treatment, such a process – for example, the authorisation of a deprivation of liberty in a hospital or residential setting – can be difficult and complex when a patient is non-cooperative with health and social care provision. There will be occasions where such a decision rests on the margins between the MHA and MCA. As Bishop (2019) notes, '…it is not always about making the "right" or "wrong" decisions, but about making evidence-based decisions in line with the law and accepted guidance…'. The defensibility of such decisions can be greatly assisted by the nurse and other clinical team members, ensuring that they document their assessment, rationale and subsequent actions.

References

Adebowale, V, 2013. Independent report: Independent Commission on Mental Health and Policing. Available at: https://www.basw.co.uk.

Barber, P, Brown, R, Martin, D, 2017. Mental health law in England & Wales: a guide for mental health professionals, 3rd ed. Sage, London.

Bishop, E, 2019. The interface between the Mental Health Act 1983 and the Mental Capacity Act 2005. Mark Allen Group Education, London. Available at. https://adults.ccinform.co.uk.

Cairns, R, Richardson, G, Hotopf, M, 2010. Deprivation of Liberty: Mental Capacity Act Safeguards versus the Mental Health Act. The Psychiatrist Online 34: 246-247. Available at: http://pb.rcpsych.org/.

Department of Health, 2015. Mental Health Act 1983: Code of practice. TSO Publications.

Department of Health and Social Care, 2018. Independent review of the Mental Health Act: interim report. Available at: https://www.gov.uk/government/groups/independent-review-of=the-mental-health-act.

Department of Health and Social Care, 2018. Modernising the Mental Health Act – increasing choice, reducing compulsion: final report from the independent review. Available at: https://www.gov.uk/government/publications/modernising-the-mental-health-act-final-report-from-the-independent-review.

Herring, J, 2020. Medical Law and Ethics (8th ed). Oxford University Press.

Lynch, RM, Simpson, M, Higson, M, Grout, P, 2002. Section 136, the Mental Health Act 1983: levels of knowledge among accident and emergency doctors, senior nurses, and police constables. Emergency Medicine Journal 19, 295–300.

Ministry of Justice, 2008. Deprivation of liberty safeguards: code of practice to supplement the main Mental Capacity Act 2005 code of practice. TSO, London. Available at: https://webarchive.nationalarchives.gov.uk.

CASES

B v Croydon Health Authority [1995] Fam 133

Clunis v Camden and Islington Health Authority [1998] QB 978.

G v E v A Local Authority v F [2010] EWHC 621 (Fam)

HL v UK Application no 45508/99 [2004] ECtHR 471

JE v DE and Surrey County Council and Others [2006] EWHC 3459 (Fam)

London Borough of Hillingdon v Neary [2011] EWHC 1377

M.S. v United Kingdom [2012] ECtHR 804

Norfolk & Norwich Healthcare (NHS) Trust v W [1996] 2 FLR 613

Nottinghamshire Healthcare NHS Trust v RC [2014] EWCOP 1317

P (by his litigation friend the Official Solicitor) (Appellant) v Cheshire West and Chester Council and another (Respondents); P and Q (by their litigation friend, the Official Solicitor) (Appellants) v Surrey County Council (Respondent) [2014] UKSC 19

Re C (An Adult: Refusal of Medical Treatment) [1994] 1 All Er 819

Re KB (Adult) (Mental Patient: Medical Treatment) [1994] 19 BMLR 144

Tameside and Glossop Acute Services Trust v CH (Patient) 1 FLR 762 (QBD)

STATUTE

Care Standards Act 2000

Human Rights Act 1998

Mental Capacity Act 2005

Mental Health Act 1983

Mental Health Act 2007

Note: Page numbers followed by "*f*" indicate figures "*t*" indicate tables and "*b*" indicate boxes.